Talking Health with
Dr. Brian
McDonough

In the series
Health, Society, and Policy,
edited by Sheryl Ruzek and Irving Kenneth Zola

TALKING HEALTH
with
Dr. Brian McDonough

Edited by

Brian P. McDonough, M.D.

Temple University Press
Philadelphia

Temple University Press, Philadelphia 19122
Copyright © 1994 by Temple University. All rights reserved
Published 1994
Printed in the United States of America

Library of Congress Cataloging-in-Publication Data

Talking health with Dr. Brian McDonough / edited by Brian P. McDonough.
    p.   cm. — (Health, society, and policy)
  ISBN 1-56639-207-1
  1. Health.   I. McDonough, Brian P., 1958–   .   II. Title: Talking
health with Doctor Brian McDonough.   III. Series.
RA776.T19   1995
613—dc20   94-6020

To my wife, Diane, and my parents.

It is their support that keeps me
striving to do more.

Contents

Foreword

Today, bookstore shelves are filled with health books for the general consumer. *Talking Health with Dr. Brian McDonough* is unique in that it was developed as a guide to preventive care and to the appropriate use of the health care system. Readers will find useful discussions of criteria for selecting health care providers, hospitals, and insurance, as well as specific information about health problems that will help them develop health-promoting life-styles.

As this book goes to press, the nation's attention is focused on the American health care system and its financial problems. One of the crucial elements in revamping our approach to health care is a recognition that preventive medicine and appropriate use of the health care system are crucial to the individual's and the nation's well-being. When we consider the history of medicine, we realize that the greatest and most cost-effective impacts on the health of populations have resulted from public health and epidemiologic advances. That is, the promotion of healthy life-styles and preventive measures have benefited humanity to a much larger degree than have dramatic changes in technology or the discovery of curative drugs. The goal of healthy living is to prevent disease entirely or to detect it at such an early stage that cure, control, or prevention of complications can be accomplished with minimal intervention by health professionals. This is also the aim of good medical practice, and it is hardly coincidental that this approach is cost-effective.

As we all know, sometimes preventive measures do not adequately protect us from disease. The information in *Talking Health with Dr. Brian McDonough* will help readers determine when a problem is clearly present and will provide advice on the appropriate use of the health care system. As a physician, I believe strongly that the key to receiving appropriate and effective health care is to select a primary care physician (that is, a family physician, general internist, general pediatrician, or an obstetrician/gynecologist) in whom you have confidence. A primary care physician is an entry point to the health care system and is a guide through it. Although the United States has an abundance of health care resources, the profusion of options can be bewildering—especially when one is under the stress of dealing with an illness. A primary care physician is trained to help patients find the most effective and efficient means to deal with their specific health problems. This book will help you select a primary care physician, and it offers basic information to help you understand the nature of specific illnesses and to assist you in making good use of the health care system.

    I can think of no better editor for a book of this sort than Brian McDonough, M.D. I have known him since he was a medical student at Temple University School of Medicine, and he is now my colleague at St. Francis Hospital. He has devoted his career to informing the public, students of medicine, and health professionals about health issues. In this book Dr. McDonough has brought together renowned experts to discuss today's most important health topics. Thus, he has produced a distinguished volume and made an important contribution to preventive medicine.

STEPHEN R. PERMUT, M.D., J.D.
Vice President for Medical Affairs
St. Francis Hospital
Wilmington, Delaware

Preface

As an outgrowth of my radio program, "Health Talk America," this book provides a basic introduction to a variety of health topics. Each chapter has been written by a leading expert on the subject; each discusses a common health problem, outlining the latest information about its causes, symptoms, treatments, and preventive measures. Each chapter includes a section in which the expert and I respond to the questions, or composites of the questions, my radio audience most often ask about the problem. Chapter 15, "Sleep Regulation for Children and Adults," is the only exception. All the answers there are provided by Dr. Getsy.

After taking calls from concerned listeners for seven years, I concluded that these frequently asked questions point to a need for nontechnical introductions to the health issues most of us encounter. Either we ourselves or members of our families experience allergies, cancers, childhood diseases, sports injuries, and so forth. Though most people have some knowledge about these health problems, few have enough information to feel confident that they are taking adequate preventive measures or that they are seeking a health provider's help early enough to avoid serious problems. For instance, people know about the general risks associated with high levels of cholesterol in foods, but they should also be familiar with the varieties of fats and oils and how they affect cholesterol levels so that they can make informed dietary choices. Similarly, people who are resolved to increase their level of physical fitness talk about building muscle, but few may recognize the value of flexibility and its role in preventing injury.

This book is intended to make such complicated topics easier to understand so that you can take greater responsibility for your own good health. It will not end your reliance on health care providers, but it may help you to develop good health practices and to use the health care system wisely. Reading it is the first step; applying its lessons will put you on the road to good health.

Many people made tremendous contributions to this book. First, I wish to thank the physicians and health experts who wrote these chapters. All of them have been guests on my radio program, and they were selected to contribute to this work because they are excellent communicators, able to make complex medical information sound simple.

I would like to thank several people who indirectly helped me put this work together. Included are Bob Stec, who helped keep "Health Talk America" on the air in its early years, and Joel Adler, who is playing a critical role as the program continues into the 1990s. I also wish to thank those who believe that a physician can also be a teacher. They have helped me achieve that goal. They include Dr. Kent Sallee, Dr. John Seydow, Roger LaMay, and Scott Herman. All are leaders in their own fields but also have a strong sense of the importance of educating the public about health.

Of course, a book of this nature cannot be written without editorial help. To this end I thank Janet Francendese and Sheryl Ruzek of Temple University Press.

Thanks to Greg Adams, M.D., and Carl J. Adams for artwork and Terry Roberts for photography.

I also want to thank Barbara Schearer for typing and retyping the chapters, and for occasionally adding the reader's perspective. There were many changes made as a result of her insight.

Finally, I thank the callers to "Health Talk America" who have asked the questions and given health care providers an idea of the major concerns of Americans when it comes to health care.

Talking Health with
Dr. Brian
McDonough

1

AIDS Risks and Testing

Marshall T. Williams, M.D., Ph.D.

The acquired immunodeficiency syndrome (AIDS) is usually a fatal disease that causes disregulation of the human immune system and is itself caused by infection with the human immunodeficiency virus (HIV). The syndrome was first described in the late 1980s, when physicians in Los Angeles, New York, and San Francisco observed an outbreak of opportunistic infections in homosexual men. About the same time, the occurrence of a fairly rare tumor (Kaposi's sarcoma) was noted in young homosexual men from the same areas. Eventually, it was found that all of these individuals suffered from an immune system defect in a particular form of white blood cell called a CD4, a T4, or "helper," lymphocyte. The fact that the affected individuals had previously been healthy strongly suggested that this defect was acquired rather than inherited or congenital. In 1982 the Centers for Disease Control established a set of criteria defining the particular syndrome. By 1983 it was found that the syndrome existed in heterosexual partners of intravenous drug users and a number of Haitians. It was not until 1983 that the agent causing AIDS was discovered and eventually found to be the virus HIV-I.

The Origin and Spread of the Disease

Until AIDS became an unmistakable plague throughout the world, the twentieth century's greatest pandemic was the Great Influenza Epidemic of 1918–1919. In its three waves of infection during that year, 549,000

1

people died in the United States; the death toll worldwide was 21 million.

The World Health Organization (WHO) estimated that by the end of 1993, between 10 million and 20 million people were infected with HIV. (These were people who had the virus; a much smaller number of people had the symptoms of AIDS.) WHO predicted that at least 30 million people around the world would be infected with HIV by 2000. Estimates have ranged as high as 110 million. Worldwide, the number of known AIDS cases is estimated at 1.7 million. The largest proportion (69 percent) has been noted in the African continent; North and South America account for about 25 percent, with 16 percent occurring in the United States. Of the remaining cases, 6 percent are in Europe, and the rest of the world combined makes up only about 1 percent. Among epidemiologists, it is well known that in Africa the disease is predominantly passed through sexual contact between heterosexuals, whereas this mode accounts for roughly 6 percent of transmission in the United States (4 percent is unknown). Some researchers have suggested that strains of HIV occurring in Africa and Thailand (where heterosexual transmission is also much more common) might be different from strains found in the United States. At present, scientists have not identified any different strains.

The increase in AIDS infections has been accompanied by a higher frequency in the appearance of other diseases. The infection rates of both syphilis and tuberculosis have been climbing remarkably. Syphilis infection rates around the world have now tripled, and tuberculosis rates have become much more alarming. The development of a multiple antibiotic-resistant strain of tuberculosis is a matter of great concern because of the threat it poses to community members and to health care providers. Tuberculosis is spread relatively easily by respiratory droplet inhalation. The severity of these worldwide problems is reflected in the high costs of current health care to WHO, whose 1992 budget is $90 million (down $20 million from 1991).

The total number of AIDS cases in the United States is approximately three hundred thousand. Two-thirds to three-fourths of those patients have already died. In the United States, HIV has shown an epidemiologic propensity to infect African Americans and Hispanic immigrants. Until recently, men had a much higher infection rate than women, but this trend has been rapidly reversing and it is estimated that by 2000 the infection rate among women will surpass that of men.

In March 1992 a rigorous debate about the origin and development of the AIDS epidemic was conducted in the pages of *Rolling Stone* and *The Lancet*. In an article entitled "The Origin of AIDS" (*Rolling Stone*, March 19, 1992), Tom Curtis proposed that oral polio vaccine contaminated with a retrovirus (the RNA-containing virus family of which HIV is a member) was used in the inoculation of three hundred thousand people in Zaire in the 1950s and that this may well have transmitted an early form of HIV. John Cohen's rebuttal to this argument was published in *Science*, August 21, 1992. He studied the epidemiologic analysis of individuals who received the vaccine but could not identify a clear path of transmission because other risk factors were present in individuals who became HIV infected. He also noted that the Wistar Institute in Philadelphia was performing HIV analyses of stored polio vaccine stock cultures. No evidence of HIV was found.

Other theories suggest that the virus may actually have begun in another form within a population of primates (monkeys) in Zaire. Researchers believe that, eventually, through mutational change, the virus was able to infect humans, possibly by being transmitted through animal bites. However, no one has been able to provide an epidemiologically adequate explanation of exactly how the virus could then have drifted into gay populations in the United States. Its origins are still unknown, but HIV has infected many people in the United States and the Third World, with devastating epidemiologic and sociologic consequences.

How HIV Infects the Body

Researchers eventually isolated HIV from the blood of individuals with AIDS, as well as from individuals who had no symptoms but who were felt to be at risk for developing the syndrome. Since that time, the virus has been isolated from other cells of the body, including bone marrow cells and certain cells found in connective tissue. The virus has a particular affinity for the "helper" lymphocyte, a member of the white blood cell family. Upon gaining access to an uninfected individual, the virus attaches itself to a certain area on the outer cell wall and then transports its genetic material (RNA) to the inside of the cell.

Once the virus has inserted itself into the host cell, it copies the cell's DNA. (DNA is the genetic controlling substance for human cells.) This transcribed, translated DNA then gains passage into the innermost portion of the human lymphocyte and eventually inserts itself into the genetic material of the host. The virus-generated DNA may sit quietly inside the host cell for many years, or it may begin making copies of itself. These copies of the virus take over the genetic and molecular factory of the lymphocyte, rendering the lymphocyte nonfunctional and eventually killing it. In that process, numerous copies of totally functional and infectious HIV particles are released, free to invade uninfected cells.

This invasion and cell destruction continues over a period of years, and the decreases in the number of the "helper" lymphocytes can be measured in a laboratory test. Normally, a person has between six hundred and one thousand "helper" lymphocytes per cubic millimeter of blood. As the disease progresses, that count may drop below two hundred. At this point the individual appears to become vulnerable to infections, such as a pneumonia caused by the parasite Pneumocystis, a meningitis caused by a fungus, Cryptococcus, or other "opportunistic" infections. The particular pathogens causing these infections are continually present in our environment and, indeed, may live inside the human body. When an HIV-infected individual's immune system deteriorates because of the continued death of the "helper" lymphocytes, these organisms are able to set up an infection, growing to the point that they destroy the person's organs. When this has occurred, the patient is said to have developed clinical AIDS.

HIV Transmission

Major epidemiologic studies show that the AIDS virus is spread in much the same way as are hepatitis B viral infections: through sexual intercourse, through intravenous (IV) drug abuse in which needles or injected drugs are shared, through transfusions, or during the growth of a fetus inside an infected mother's womb. The exact portal of entry of the viral infection has yet to be identified.

It is important to emphasize how AIDS is *not* spread. No one has yet been shown to have been infected through working with an AIDS patient or living in the home of an AIDS patient. Many epidemiologic studies have been done that look at whether people living in the same home as an HIV-infected person become infected. The studies thus far have shown that only individuals who are sexual partners of the infected patient or who share a common risk factor (such as intravenous drug abuse) typically become infected. Other people living in the home or helping the patient have not been shown to become infected (through a recent description of a sibling of an HIV-infected child contracting the virus has challenged this notion.) People who give blood do not become infected. Blood is drawn with sterile instruments that have not been exposed to humans; therefore, donating blood presents no risk whatsoever of acquiring or transmitting the disease. Nonetheless, people's fear of contracting AIDS is felt to be a contributing factor to considerable shortage of blood supplies in many areas.

People frequently ask if AIDS has been shown to be transmitted by a nonhuman living organism. Malaria, for example, is a parasite known to be carried from person to person by the Anopheles mosquito, which bites an infected person and then transmits the parasite to an uninfected person. Similarly, the deer tick acquires the Lyme bacteria by feeding on infected deer. It then transmits this bacteria by biting an unsuspecting person. Some large-scale epidemiologic studies have monitored the number of mosquito bites in an endemic area and then looked at the relative frequency of HIV conversion on blood tests. Although the number of bites remains the same among children, the elderly, and individuals at risk for HIV disease, neither the children nor the elderly have shown an increased rate of infection. Only individuals who had a known risk (such as intravenous drug abuse) were infected with HIV. These results rule out a potential nonhuman transmission source.

Women's Risks

In Africa, where heterosexual transmission predominates, epidemiologic studies paint a frightening picture of the extent of the infection. In Zaire over four million people in the capital city of Kinshasa are believed to be HIV-positive (roughly 7 percent of the population). Some 18 percent of all blood donors in Zambia are known to be HIV-positive, and one estimate suggests that 67 percent of all street prostitutes in Nairobi, Kenya, are HIV-positive. Some of the most startling numbers come out of urban Rwanda; in a 1991 study of nearly fifteen hundred childbearing women between ages nineteen and thirty-seven, 32 percent were found to have evidence of infection with HIV. The incidence was higher in single women, but even of those who were in a monogamous relationship, 20 percent were infected with the virus.

These numbers have raised very important issues regarding the infection in women throughout the world:

- Eighty percent to 85 percent of HIV-infected women are in their child-bearing years. (Fifty-one percent of HIV-infected women are IV drug abusers, 30 percent are heterosexual contacts of a man who is known to be infected, 11 percent have been infected through blood transfusions, and about 7 percent have been infected by undetermined routes).

- Male-to-female transmission may be ten times higher than the female-to-male rate. The reasons for this are unknown, but such factors as vaginal trauma, intrauterine contraceptive devices, and genital ulceration by other infectious agents may be involved. In Western culture, the vaginal spermicide nonoxynol-9, which has been touted as an aid to safer sex, is also known to cause cervical inflammation, which may provide an irritated vaginal surface that permits easier transmission of the viral infection.

- The presenting symptoms of AIDS in women are still the same as those in men. Pneumonia with the parasite *Pneumocystis carinii* is still the most opportunistic infection. Women have been noted to have a higher incidence of fungal infections of the esophagus, however. Many experts have considered that chronic infections found in women at other sites (such as chronic vaginitis) might also be early indicators of HIV or AIDS infection.

- Women appear to die earlier in the course of the disease than do men. Specifically, of all the patients who have been diagnosed as having AIDS, 59 percent of the women have already died as opposed to 50 percent of the men. Speculations about the reasons for this discrepancy in the death rate involve the factors of early misdiagnosis of HIV infection; delay of women entering the medical care process; exclusion of women, particularly of childbearing age, from possible treatment; and the question of the reliability of condoms for protection against HIV infection. Numerous studies have shown that condoms may fail to prevent pregnancy 15 percent to 18 percent of the time. The HIV particle is roughly four hundred times smaller than a human sperm.

Indeed, women present an entire spectrum of issues unique to their sex. In HIV disease there is known to be an increased incidence of gynecologic disease: pelvic inflammatory disease (PID), abscesses of the pelvic cavity, and human papilloma virus (HPV), which causes warts in the genital area and is known to be associated with cervical cancer. HPV infection is believed to affect between 2 percent and 15 percent of HIV-negative women and between 25 percent and 95 percent of HIV-positive women. Therefore, HIV-infected women are expected to have a three- to tenfold higher rate of abnormal Pap smears. Indeed, 85 percent of HIV-infected women have abnormal cervical visual exams (colposcopies), and 41 percent of these have cervical intraepithelial neoplasia, which are abnormal cells on or near the cervix.

Similarly, HIV also raises many obstetric issues. In one study of HIV-infected pregnant women, only 17 percent entered prenatal care in their first trimester. Mother-to-child transmission rates have been studied in depth and range between 20 percent and 35 percent. It has been shown that if the infection actually takes place in the later stages of pregnancy, the rate of HIV-positive offspring increases. The reason for this may be that, during pregnancy in noninfected women, the number of "helper" lymphocytes drops to a nadir at the thirty-second week and then rises rapidly just before delivery. In HIV-infected women, a similar pattern is seen, but the swings are more accentuated. This fluctuation might explain the rapid progression of HIV disease seen during pregnancy.

Teenagers' Risks

One measure of HIV infection among teenagers is provided by U.S. military data, because all applicants to the military are tested. Infection rates have been running at roughly one in every twenty-five hundred to three thousand applicants and are similar for men and women. The rate of infection in African American applicants, however, is three times higher. Indeed, in urban counties in the northeastern United States, the rate was greater than one in five hundred applicants. In the northern central United States, it was less than one in ten thousand applicants. These figures follow demographic guidelines that show higher incidences of HIV infections, in general, in the northeastern and the more highly populated corridors of the United States. Other epidemiologic surveys have predicted that between one in three hundred and one in five hundred college students may be infected with HIV.

These rates are most alarming when one looks at data showing increased sexual activity among teenagers. A large study carried out in Canada in 1990 looked at over five thousand college freshmen and found that by age nineteen 74 percent of all males and almost 69 percent of all females had had intercourse. Approximately 15 percent were engaging in anal intercourse, which is believed to have a higher incidence of transmission of HIV. Over 20 percent of the men and 8 percent of the women had already had more than ten partners by age nineteen. Having multiple partners is similarly believed to increase the risk of HIV infection. Only 21 percent of the men and 7.5 percent of the women regularly used condoms; nonusers cited multiple partners, embarrassment in purchasing condoms, inability to discuss condom use with their partner, insufficient knowledge of sexually transmitted diseases, and an expected decrease in pleasure as reasons they avoided condoms. A large percentage of the women stated a preference for oral contraceptives, totally missing the point that they were not protected against sexually transmitted disease without the use of a barrier method of contraception.

Even young teens are sexually active. A study reported by the Centers for Disease Control in April 1992 noted that one in eight high school freshmen had already had more than four sexual partners, and that by the time the same group became seniors, one in four had already had more than four partners. This activity clearly appears to correlate with the increased incidence of all sexually transmitted diseases in the very young. About ten million to twenty million cases of sexually transmitted diseases occur annually in the United States, and 65 percent of these occur in individuals who are less than twenty-five years old. It is not surprising, then, that teenagers are especially vulnerable to the AIDS epidemic.

It is clear that we need new antiviral chemotherapy to treat those already infected. In addition, we need better preventive measures, aimed at protecting those individuals at risk for the disease. As part of those preventive measures, there needs to be effective prevention of the transmission of the virus between sexual partners. Though barrier contraception and chemical inactivation of the virus offer some level of protection, public health efforts must focus on decreasing the number of sexual partners, particularly among younger individuals (who appear to be less likely to use barrier protection). Furthermore, we should develop a concept of sexual reform that encourages young people to move away from intercourse as a means of expressing their caring needs.

Testing for HIV

As with most infections, a person develops antibodies to the HIV infection. With some diseases, antibodies protect the individual from infection, but this is *not* true with HIV (or syphilis or tuberculosis). The presence of antibodies does indicate, however, that the person has been infected. The antibody to HIV develops roughly six to eight weeks after the person first becomes infected (whether by needle stick, infected wound, intercourse, or blood transfusion) and can be detected by any one of several different techniques.

If an individual has two positive screening tests (the Elisa or EIA test) for the antibody, a confirmatory test called a Western Blot is performed to look for the antibody to the various components of the virus. If this test is also positive, the individual is informed that he or she has indeed had a positive test for the antibody to HIV disease, indicating that the person is infected with the virus. Individuals so infected will likely develop AIDS. Note, however, that up to 70 percent of initially positive *screening tests* for HIV are negative on the second, more accurate, diagnostic test (the Western Blot). The need for counseling is great. People being tested for HIV need to feel that they have support and are not isolated. Clearly, there is more to the HIV test than a positive or negative result, and people must feel that help is available throughout the process. The current recommendations from the Centers for Disease Control are that the following individuals should seek HIV screening tests:

- homosexual or bisexual males active *even once* since 1977
- intravenous drug abusers
- prostitutes and their partners
- people with symptoms suggestive of AIDS

About the Author

Dr. Marshall T. Williams is a specialist in the field of infectious disease. He received his M.D. and his Ph.D. in microbiology from the University of Rochester, New York.

Dr. Williams performed his residency at the Bowman Gray School of Medicine and his infectious disease fellowship at Walter Reed Army Medical Center. He is now in private practice in Wilmington, Delaware, and on the teaching staff of the Medical Center of Delaware and St. Francis Hospital.

QUESTIONS FOR THE DOCTOR

Q: HIV *is gaining a great deal of attention as a sexually transmitted disease. What about other diseases? Isn't syphilis making a comeback?*

A: Yes. In fact it has been making a strong comeback since about 1985. The cause has not changed; the spirochete *Treponema pallidum* has caused the disease for generations. Penicillin is the classic treatment for all stages of syphilis, but other medications and antibiotics can also be quite effective. The problem is that many cases of syphilis are not diagnosed. Despite its comeback, many doctors have not seen cases of syphilis and are not certain of the symptoms.

On average, twenty-one days pass before signs of syphilis are evident, but the range can be ten to ninety days. The classic lesion is a *chancre,* a button-like spot that can develop into a painless erosion and later form an ulcer with a raised border. The chancre is red and firm, often described as "meaty" colored, and the border is darker than the rest of it. Because the chancre is painless, people often ignore it. That can be a serious mistake. Early diagnosis and treatment are necessary to avoid the development of later stages of syphilis, which can severely affect the heart and nervous system. HIV infection seems to predispose a syphilis patient to a more serious course of infection, and syphilis seems to increase the probability of acquiring HIV.

Q: *I had a pelvic inflammatory disease two years ago, which my doctor treated with an antibiotic. Could having this disease be any risk for me in the future?*

A: *Pelvic inflammatory disease* (PID) is a medical term that includes a wide variety of problems with the female reproductive system, including infections of the lining of the uterus, infections of the Fallopian tubes or the ovaries, and even an infection called a *peritonitis.* These problems should be taken seriously. Scarring from pelvic infections that have not been properly treated is one of the leading causes of infertility. Roughly 25 percent of women with PID become infertile. Bacteria such as *N. gonorrhea* and *Chlamydia trachomatis* may cause PID. Your health care provider must perform an internal gynecologic examination to tell if you have a pelvic infection. Women may also have to have an examination with an instrument called a *laparoscope* and have cultures done to check for the cause of infection. The symptoms of a pelvic infection include fever, chills, back pain on one or both sides, and a discharge. If you are experiencing any of these problems, you should consult your doctor.

This is a serious illness, but if PID is diagnosed early enough and if it is properly treated, you should have little to be concerned about in terms of future problems.

Q: *Can a sexually transmitted disease cause eye irritation?*

A: Yes, a number of sexually transmitted diseases, including *gonorrhea* and *chlamydia,* may cause problems or infections in the eyes. If your gynecologist's treatment for the sexually transmitted disease is not effective in curing your eye problems, or if they appear to be serious, he or she will refer you to an ophthalmologist for further evaluation.

Q: *I am a man and have been suffering from pain on urination, eye pain, and a great deal of pain in my knee and index finger where the joint is. Am I falling apart?*

A: Doctors cannot diagnose someone properly without a physical exam, but your symptoms might be related to *Reiter's syndrome,* which can cause inflammation of the tube inside the penis (called the urethra), eye inflammation, and arthritis. Reiter's syndrome can be caused by chlamydia, a sexually transmitted organism, but not all cases have been sexually transmitted; in fact, there have been cases of Reiter's that have been shown to be related to epidemic dysentery. The number of cases of Reiter's syndrome has also been found to be increased in people with HIV infection. (Many illnesses can be made worse by an existing infection with HIV.) You should see your doctor to find out what is causing your symptoms.

Q: *We know how AIDS is spread. What are some of the ways that have been ruled out?*

A: HIV infection is not known to be caused by close personal contact. Also, it does not spread by people living in the same household, workplace, or school, unless they share needles or have sexual contact. A recent report of possible infection between siblings remains to be clarified. HIV infection is very difficult to get by the routes that commonly cause the spread of most viruses.

Q: *My friend said that I can get AIDS from donating blood. Is there any risk of this?*

A: No. There is no risk of contracting HIV from donating blood. This is one of the misconceptions surrounding the AIDS virus. Unfortunately, this misconception has had the dramatic effect of lowering the amount of donated blood available for people to use in cases of emergency.

Q: *I have heard that AIDS is an inner-city disease. Is this true?*

A: AIDS is a disease that can affect anyone, anywhere, at any time. Some of the fallacies that have led to difficulty in treating this disease are that AIDS is a disease that affects only poor people in the inner city or that AIDS attacks only male homosexuals. At the present time in the United States, the incidence of AIDS is more than three times higher among African Americans and Hispanics than among whites, and most white patients are either homosexual or bisexual. However, as the number of people with AIDS has increased, so has its transmission. Many researchers are frightened about the heterosexual spread of HIV, including that in young people who fail to listen to many of the reports concerning safe sex.

Q: *If I use a condom every time I have sexual intercourse, am I protected from HIV?*
A: You are more protected than if you do not use a condom. You may still get the virus, however, because condoms are not 100 percent effective. The only 100 percent effective method of not getting HIV is abstinence. It is important to remember that condoms are better than nothing, but they are far from perfect. Women can get pregnant even though condoms are used, and it is foolish to think that women and men cannot get HIV, even though they are using a barrier method of protection.

Q: *My doctor diagnosed me with* Trichomonas. *What is this?*
A: *Trichomonas* is a sexually transmitted disease. Doctors are often able to make the diagnosis by taking a culture during a gynecologic exam and then seeing the offending agent spinning around on the slide under a microscope. A woman with trichomonas may notice vaginal secretions, pain on urination, and a foul-smelling discharge, which is usually yellow-green. It is relatively easy for doctors to diagnose trichomonas, and it can be treated quite effectively with antibiotics; however, as with all sexually transmitted diseases, it is critical that your partner also be treated. If not, you will be passing the disease back and forth.

Q: *My doctor says I have a* candida *infection. My friend said that this is a sexually transmitted disease, but I haven't had a partner in over two years. Do you think I have candida?*
A: *Candida* is a yeast infection, and there is no absolute link to sexual contact. In other words, you do not have to have intercourse to get a yeast infection. Some people are more prone to these problems because they are diabetics or have an altered immune system for one of many reasons. Taking oral contraceptives may make someone more likely to get yeast infections, and many pregnant women get these infections. The most common symptoms of candida infection are itchiness in the vaginal area and the presence of a whitish discharge that looks like cottage cheese. Treatment is simple. In fact, women now are using many over-the-counter medications. However, be cautious about failing to go to your doctor when you are experiencing vaginal infections, because unless you are certain that what you have is a yeast infection, you could actually be delaying diagno-

sis of a more serious sexually transmitted disease. As I mentioned earlier, serious infections can interfere with fertility and pregnancy.

Q: My partner has warts on his penis. Can he spread these to me?

A: It is not only possible but also quite probable. These warts are caused by the *human papilloma virus* (HPV). Depending on what type of papilloma virus your partner has, his exposing you to this infectious agent could increase your chances of having cancer of the cervix later in life. Genital warts can often be seen on close inspection, but many times they are microscopic and can only be detected by a Pap smear. Large visible warts can be treated by a number of methods, including cryosurgery, which uses freezing to kill the cells. However, once you are exposed to this virus, it can recur throughout life. Human papilloma virus infection is an epidemic and, without doubt, is one of the most common sexually transmitted diseases.

If you have a history of HPV and see your gynecologist for Pap smears every year, there is a good chance that cervical cancer, if it were to occur, can be detected and treated. One final point: although the rate of cervical cancer is increased in women with HPV, this cancer occurs rarely. I want you to be concerned but not afraid.

Q: What is the most common sexually transmitted disease?

A: Each year in the United States there are three million to four million cases of chlamydia infection, two million cases of gonorrhea, and thirty-five thousand cases of primary and secondary syphilis. A new onset of *Herpes simplex* infection occurs in 207,000 Americans every year. Twenty million people are already infected and suffering recurrent episodes of herpes. I mentioned that HPV is becoming the most common sexually transmitted disease, but the rate of infection is far more difficult to measure because the virus is usually microscopic and the disease is diagnosed only in a culture. Another major concern is hepatitis B, which is spread primarily through the exchange of blood and blood products. Five hundred thousand to one million Americans have been infected with hepatitis B virus. Chronic carriers of hepatitis B virus are at risk for developing chronic active hepatitis, cirrhosis, and even liver cancer. As many as five thousand people die each year as a result of these complications.

HIV and AIDS are personally frightening and are a major health problem, but their existence should not cause people to underestimate these other sexually transmitted diseases. They, too, can be devastating.

Q: What is the proper way to use a condom?

A: According to the *Guide to Clinical Preventive Services,* a report of the United States Preventive Services Task Force, men should use latex condoms, rather than natural membrane condoms (such as lamb-skin). Torn condoms, those in damaged packages, or those with signs of age (brittle, sticky, or discolored) should not be used. The condom should be put on an erect penis before any intimate contact and should be unrolled completely to the base. A space should be left at the tip of the condom to collect semen, and air pockets in this space should be removed by pressing the air outward toward the base.

Only water-based lubricants should be used. Those made with petroleum jelly, mineral oil, cold cream, or other oil-based products should *not* be applied because they may damage the condom. Insertion of nonoxynol-9 in the condom increases protection, but vaginal application of this spermicide, in addition to condom use, will provide greater protection against pregnancy and disease. Be aware, however, that a new study has shown that nonoxynol-9 can add to vaginal irritation, and openings in the vaginal walls from abrasion may add to a possible risk of infection.

If a condom breaks, it should be replaced immediately. After ejaculation and while the penis is still erect, the penis should be withdrawn while carefully holding the condom against the base of the penis so that the condom remains in place. The condom should not be reused. Once again, I want to emphasize that condoms are not 100 percent effective, and as new studies become available, we are learning about other potential problems associated with them. However, using them is far better than not using them. A female condom is now available, and although not enough data are yet available for us to make a conclusive statement, its use can help women protect themselves against both pregnancy and sexually transmitted diseases.

2

Breast and Gynecologic Cancers

Robert C. Young, M.D.

This year more than 500,000 American women will learn that they have cancer. Cancer is the leading killer of American women between ages forty and seventy. This chapter deals primarily with cancers that affect female organs—breast, ovarian, cervical, and endometrial cancers—but it is important to remember that women get other cancers as well.

Until the early 1960s, lung cancer was relatively rare in women, mostly because women did not start smoking in large numbers until the early 1940s. Since then, lung cancer has become the fastest-rising cancer among women; the number of new cases and deaths has risen steadily and continues to rise. Lung cancer has now passed breast cancer as the leading cancer killer of women, with more than fifty thousand deaths a year. Also among the most common cancers in women are cancers of the colon and rectum, cancer of the uterus, ovarian cancer, and lymphoma (which affects the lymphatic system).

Breast Cancer

Scarcely a month goes by without news reports, personal stories, or advice about some aspect of *breast cancer* appearing in print or broadcast media. Some term this disease epidemic. It affects more women in this country than any other cancer, with an estimated 182,000 new cases a year and 46,000 deaths annually, according to the American Cancer

15

Society. Awareness of the threat of breast cancer has never been higher. Although that knowledge can generate anxiety, the constant publicity about breast cancer has helped to change the way women view their interactions with the health care system and has fueled the drive to gain more control over breast cancer through early detection and treatment choices.

Many women fear breast cancer. It has a major psychological impact, threatening not only a woman's life but also her self-image and sexuality. Often the first thought on diagnosis is "Will I die?"; the second is "Will I lose my breast?"

For most women today, the answer to both questions is no. Improvements in the detection and treatment of breast cancer have increased both survival rates and the quality of life for patients. Overall, the five-year survival rate is about 65 percent. For women with early disease, that rate increases to more than 90 percent. The majority of women with breast cancer can be treated with limited surgery, removing only the lump and surrounding tissue, followed by radiation therapy. The result in many women is an almost normal-appearing breast.

There are reasons to be optimistic about breast cancer treatment, but areas of concern remain. Although it is often possible to treat women with recurrent breast cancer successfully for many years, no truly curative therapies exist once the disease has spread. Too many women, especially poor and medically underserved women, are still being diagnosed with advanced disease, and their survival rates are much lower. Treatment approaches in different regions of the country continue to vary, for reasons that have nothing to do with good medicine. A breast cancer patient in the South, for example, is far more likely to have a mastectomy than is a patient in the Northeast.

We also need to know more about the genetic and environmental factors that influence breast cancer development, and we need convincing studies to test new ways to prevent this cancer. Its incidence appears to be rising, and all the reasons are not clear.

Much has been said about the risk factors for breast cancer. Overall, a white American woman has approximately a one in eight risk of getting breast cancer during her lifetime. (The risk is somewhat lower for African American, Hispanic, and Asian women.) Although the overall risk is widely cited, it is a little misleading because it relies on a number of assumptions that are not true for individual women. First, it assumes that all women will live to age eighty-seven, and, second, that all women begin with the same risk of breast cancer. The net result is that one in eight overestimates the risk for women with no risk factors and underestimates it for those with risk factors.

The greatest risk of getting breast cancer stems simply from getting older. The incidence increases steadily from a very low risk at age thirty to a much higher one at age eighty. Only one-third of breast cancers occur in women younger than fifty.

Family history can also be a significant risk factor for breast cancer. By family history, we mean first-degree relatives—mothers, sisters, and daughters—who have had breast cancer. Current estimates are that only about 5 percent of all breast cancers are truly genetic, meaning that a "breast cancer gene" is passed from one generation to the next. The Margaret Dyson Family-Risk Assessment Program at Fox Chase Cancer Center in Philadelphia, Pennsylvania, sees women from these families. One woman's mother and three of her mother's sisters all died of breast cancer, beginning with the oldest and moving in order down to the youngest. Now breast cancer is beginning to occur in the next generation as well. This woman's own sister has already been diagnosed. With this family history, she herself has an enormously high risk of getting breast cancer, so she enrolled in the national Breast Cancer Prevention Trial that began in 1992. Her story, however, is relatively unusual.

A woman may also have a slightly increased risk of breast cancer if she began to menstruate before age twelve or did not reach menopause until after age fifty-five. Some researchers believe that the key factor is the total number of years a woman menstruates, with the breast cancer risk increasing after forty menstruating years.

The age at which a woman has her first full-term pregnancy also influences breast cancer risk. If every woman had a baby before age twenty, the number of breast cancers might fall by as much as 20 percent. That, of course, is not a recommendation for early motherhood, because the decision of when and whether to have children is a complex one.

It is true, however, that women who have their first child after age thirty or who never have a full-term pregnancy do have a slightly increased risk of getting breast cancer. One possible explanation for this is that between a woman's first menstrual period and her first pregnancy, breast tissue is particularly sensitive to cancer-causing agents. We do not know exactly what all of these agents are, but they likely include diet, alcohol, tobacco, radiation, and hormones.

A great deal of scientific interest has focused on the role of dietary fat in promoting breast cancer. Studies to date have yielded no clear answers about the extent of danger from a high-fat diet. A relationship seems to exist between a high-fat diet and breast cancer, but no one is sure whether other genetic factors influence the level of risk. There are, however, a lot of other good reasons for eating less fat.

Another subject of concern and study is the question of whether long-term use of hormones, either as contraceptives or as estrogen-replacement therapy after menopause, affects a woman's risk of breast cancer. Studies over the past twenty years have been confusing and contradictory, but the most recent data seem to suggest a modest increase in risk among long-term users (more than seven years), particularly in those with a family history of breast cancer.

Concerning both contraceptive and postmenopausal hormone use, the single most important thing for a woman and her physician to keep in mind is her overall health industry, including family history. These studies are not definitive, however, because of differences in contraceptive pills. Those introduced in the 1960s contained much higher hormone doses than do current birth control pills.

At the same time, research has clearly shown that oral contraceptives help to lower the risk of ovarian and endometrial cancers—a protection that appears to persist for at least fifteen years after a woman stops taking the pill. Estrogen-replacement therapy, in contrast, increases the risk of endometrial cancer. This risk of cancer of the uterine lining rises in direct proportion to how strong the hormone dose is and how long the woman takes it.

Estrogen therapy's effect on breast cancer risk has become clearer as a result of a 1991 analysis by the Centers for Disease Control, based on sixteen breast cancer studies in the United States and around the world. The CDC found that when women with a family history of breast cancer took replacement estrogen for even a short time, they more than tripled their risk of this cancer. Women without a family history of breast cancer who took estrogen for five years or less had on additional risk. Those taking it for fifteen years or more increased their risk of breast cancer by 30 percent (or by 100 percent if they began the hormone therapy during the premenopausal stage). For many women, these risks may be balanced by the potential benefits of estrogen replacement in preventing bone loss and heart disease.

Women sometimes want to know how much their risk of breast cancer is increased if they have more than one common risk factor—say, early menstruation and late pregnancy. The interaction of risk factors is a tricky and complicated issue, but it does not appear to be a matter of simple arithmetic. If you have one risk factor that increases your risk by 20 percent and one that increases your risk by 10 percent, it does not necessarily add up to 30 percent. And the vast majority of women with breast cancer—80 percent of all cases—have no known risk factors other than advancing age.

Breast Cancer Prevention

The best way to control any disease is, of course, to prevent it. The first nationwide attempt to prevent breast cancer aims to enroll more than sixteen thousand women in a randomized clinical trial, designed to determine if the drug tamoxifen can reduce breast cancer among women at high risk of the disease. Randomized means that half the participating women will receive the drug while the other half will get an inactive substance, called a placebo. All the women will receive frequent check-ups, mammograms, and access to counseling throughout the trial, which started in 1992 and will run for at least seven years.

Tamoxifen has been available for about twenty years as a treatment for diagnosed breast cancer. Researchers observed that women who got this drug as therapy following primary surgery did not develop the expected number of second cancers in the other breast. Tamoxifen blocks the cells from using estrogen, which some cancer cells need to grow. The theory and the hope is that the drug will prevent cancer from developing in the first place.

Women who participate in this trial must have a significantly higher-than-average risk of getting breast cancer. Most clinical trials are done with patients who are already sick. A prevention trial is done, by definition, with healthy people. For this reason, it becomes even more important to make sure that the potential benefits outweigh the possible risks. A level of risk acceptable to women with a life-threatening disease may not be acceptable to still-healthy women.

Clinicians have a lot of experience with tamoxifen and have found that its side effects are generally either minor or rare. The most common problem is that some women have menopausal symptoms, including hot flashes. Much less common are liver problems, uterine cancers, and eye problems. On the positive side, there is some evidence that tamoxifen protects women against osteoporosis and lowers cholesterol levels.

It will be a very important scientific advancement if tamoxifen really does lower the incidence of breast cancer. The Breast Cancer Prevention Trial will help answer that critical question. Women who are interested in participating need to be well informed about the possible risks of taking tamoxifen, but they also need to be aware of the enormous potential benefits and of the contribution this trial will make to understanding breast cancer. Regardless of whether tamoxifen works as a preventive agent, there are certain to be more trials of methods to prevent breast cancer and other major cancers. These efforts are likely to change the way we think about cancer and other diseases as well.

Genetic research in laboratories around the country will help physicians target prevention therapies to those at highest risk. Researchers are working to pinpoint the gene or genes involved in breast cancer. Inherited defects in these genes appear to be responsible for strong family histories of the disease. Nonhereditary defects in the same genes may account for many other breast cancers in women without known risk factors. Once these genes are identified, we can improve screening. A blood test may then allow a woman to know her own risk and to receive the kind of screening she needs. Eventually it may even become possible to fix these broken genes by adjusting, repairing, or replacing their cellular products.

Breast Cancer Detection

Breast cancer does not just appear one day. This disease usually takes years to develop from the first malignant cells to a tumor that can be detected by *mammography*, or breast X rays, and then to one that can be detected by physical examination. Most experts estimate that the average breast cancer is present for eight years before a mammogram can detect it and for ten years before it can be felt. Not all breast cancers are average, however. Very aggressive ones grow and spread very quickly, and others are indolent and grow very slowly.

Understanding a little about the natural history of breast cancer, how it grows and spreads, is important to the understanding of its detection and treatment.

If breast cancers remained confined to the breast, virtually no one would ever die of this disease. Cancers kill because they have the ability to metastasize—to spread to other sites in the body. The goal of cancer screening and detection programs is to detect a malignancy in its earliest stages, before it has had the chance to spread. In general, the bigger a tumor, the longer it has been present and the more likely it is to metastasize.

With this information, it is easy to see why mammography is such an important development in breast cancer screening and detection. A *mammogram* is simply an X ray of the breast that can detect a cancer as small as one-half centimeter in diameter—about the size of a small pea. Sometimes mammograms even detect precancerous conditions, tiny abnormalities of cells that have not become truly cancerous.

If every woman older than age forty would follow recommended screening guidelines and get regular mammograms, the death rate from breast cancer would fall by at least one-third. That means we would save the lives of more than fifteen thousand women a year in this country alone. Many more breast cancers would be detected early, when treatment is more successful and less difficult to undergo.

Recently, the forty-to-fifty age group has undergone greater study concerning the value of mammography, but remember that screening mammograms are done for women who have no symptoms of any kind. At *any age,* if you have a lump or other symptoms, such as abnormal discharge or thickening of the breast, you need to see your doctor right away. Don't wait until your next scheduled examination.

Despite the overwhelming evidence that mammography screening saves lives, many women do not take advantage of this procedure. Only about 60 percent of all eligible women have ever had a mammogram, and only about 40 percent get regular mammograms. Why? Studies indicate that women are far more likely to get mammograms if their own doctors recommend them. If your doctor does not talk to you about mammography once you reach age forty, you should ask about it or consider getting a new doctor.

The cost of mammograms has been an obstacle for many women in the past. For many years, insurance companies routinely refused to reimburse women for their screening mammograms. A number of states, including Pennsylvania and New Jersey, have addressed that issue by passing legislation that requires insurers to pay for screening mammography. Medicare also covers it. For many women who are not insured and who do not have the money for mammography, a number of groups—including cancer centers, the American Cancer Society, various health departments, and others—have initiated programs to provide low-cost or free mammograms. Still, too many women do not have access to affordable mammography.

Some women fear that a mammogram will hurt. The breast needs to be tightly compressed to get the best X-ray images. For most women, the procedure is much more likely to feel awkward and uncomfortable than painful. A few women with extremely sensitive breasts may feel pain and should be especially careful to schedule the exam after, rather than just before or during, their menstrual period, when their breasts are most tender. The great majority of women do not view the short-term discomfort as a deterrent to getting additional mammograms.

Finally, the major reason women avoid mammography screening is that when you're feeling fine and have no symptoms, it is hard to seek out a procedure that just might show you have a serious disease. In its early stages, breast cancer rarely causes any problems—no sickness, no pain, and no obvious lump.

Remember that nine of every ten mammograms are normal and that if something is wrong, more than 90 percent of early breast cancers can be cured, often without losing a breast. Yes, breast cancer is scary—but it won't go away if you ignore it. The later a cancer is diagnosed, the lower the odds of successful treatment. If you are scared of getting a mammogram, find a friend to go with you. That source of support makes it hard to back out at the last minute. Think about the other people in your life who depend on you and need you to do everything you can to stay healthy.

Where should you get a mammogram? The simplest answer is a facility accredited by the American College of Radiology. This will ensure that you get your examination done on good equipment by well-trained staff. You should also seek out a facility where you can ask questions of both the technologists and the radiologists.

If your mammogram is abnormal, the physician usually recommends additional tests to evaluate the problem. These will frequently include a biopsy. Most biopsies can be done on an outpatient basis, using a needle to withdraw tissue or fluid. In some instances, the surgeon will have to remove the entire lump. Then a pathologist examines the cells under the microscope to determine whether they are cancerous.

Although there have been some recent studies questioning the life-saving value of mammograms for women under age fifty, the National Cancer Institute still regards mammography as a crucial part of every women's health plan once she reaches age fifty. Mammography, however, is not perfect. Even the most sophisticated equipment can miss up to 15 percent of breast cancers. These are usually lumps at the edge of the breast and are not seen on the X-ray film. In young women, denser breast tissue makes it harder to see abnormalities.

That is why it is also important for women to practice breast self-examination and get annual breast examinations from their physicians. Mammography does not replace these two critical ways of helping to protect against breast cancer. Even some lumps that can be felt cannot be seen on mammograms. Though breast cancer is rare among women in their twenties, that is still a good age to learn breast self-examination and to begin doing it monthly, especially if a woman has a family history of the disease.

Primary Treatment for Breast Cancer

As early as the 1940s, a very few researchers had begun to question the need for radical mastectomies in treating women with breast cancer, and by the late 1960s a number of investigators were advocating more conservative, less disfiguring, approaches to breast cancer treatment. The change in approach was based on a new understanding of how breast cancers grow and spread.

The really important prognostic indicators are the size of the tumor and the number of underarm lymph nodes to which the cancer has spread. A very small tumor with no involved lymph nodes had the best prognosis. The higher the number of cancerous lymph nodes discovered, the higher the likelihood that the breast cancer has become systemic, meaning that cancer cells have migrated to other parts of the body.

For most women with breast cancer, removing the entire breast and underlying muscle is unnecessary and does not improve the chances of curing the disease. The evidence is now conclusive that we can achieve the same cure rate for breast cancer by removing only the cancerous part of the breast, a procedure known as *lumpectomy*. To ensure that all the cancer cells in the breast area have been destroyed, doctors usually recommend that a woman receive a course of radiation therapy following this surgery. The axillary (armpit) lymph nodes are usually removed at the same time so that the pathologist can examine them to determine whether the cancer has spread; knowing that is important in order to decide on the right follow-up treatment.

Please note the caveat here. Some women still need mastectomies, which includes the surgical removal of the breast and sometimes the underlying tissue, and some women choose them. Large or bulky tumors cannot be removed with a lumpectomy, nor can tumors that have invaded the chest wall. Some women prefer more extensive surgery rather than radiation therapy for five or six weeks. Lots of factors go into making decisions about the right treatment approach for each woman. The important thing, though, is that women *do* have choices. They should participate in the decisions about their treatment. Gone are the days when a woman wakes up from a breast biopsy to find that she has undergone a radical mastectomy.

You should keep two important points in mind. First, the diagnosis of cancer produces a sense of urgency. People feel that they must act immediately—that days, even hours, are crucial. But in most cases, that just is not so. You do have time to get a second opinion, to consider your options, and to understand your disease and its treatment. You should not wait for months, but you can wait for days or even several weeks without damaging your chance of recovery.

The second point is that with many cancers, and breast cancer is one of them, you need to get an opinion from a multidisciplinary team of specialists: a group including a surgeon, a radiation therapist, a medical oncologist, and often a pathologist. The team might also include a social worker or psychologist to make recommendations on the psychosocial impact of the disease.

Most cancer centers now offer consultations with a multidisciplinary breast cancer evaluation team. Regardless of where you decide to be treated, you should get an opinion from one of these groups. This helps assure that your treatment will represent the most up-to-date approach available.

Systemic Treatment for Breast Cancer

The goal of all cancer treatment is to eliminate the disease effectively while doing the least amount of damage to the patient. The more we understand about the biological nature of cancer—the way cancer cells grow, the differences between normal and cancerous cells, and the mechanisms that allow cancer cells to spread throughout the body—the better the chances of meeting this goal.

Breast cancer treatment is a good example of how cancer treatment has changed and improved during the past twenty years. More conservative treatment has allowed most women to keep their breasts and to avoid the discomfort and dysfunction caused by removing the underlying muscle. The challenge now is to develop better treatments for more aggressive breast cancers and for those that have already spread to other parts of the body. Treatments that affect the whole body rather than just one area are called *systemic treatments.*

Chemotherapy and hormonal therapy are the main systemic therapies used to treat breast cancer. Systemic therapy can be given either to try to prevent recurrence or to treat patients for cancer that has recurred.

If a woman has had surgery for her breast cancer and the pathologist finds that the cancer has spread to one or more lymph nodes under her arm, the oncologist will usually recommend additional treatment, called *adjuvant therapy,* as a preventive measure. The spread to the lymph nodes makes it likely that cancer cells remain in the body and will multiply to form a new tumor at some time in the future. It makes good sense to start the treatment soon after surgery, when the number of remaining cancer cells is probably at its lowest, so the treatment has the best chance to succeed. Oncologists have been using adjuvant therapy for breast cancer since the mid-1960s, and it has proven very effective in preventing or delaying recurrences.

About 90 percent of women with very early breast cancer can be cured with surgery and radiation alone. As mentioned, however, certain breast cancers, which doctors call "bad actors," spread rapidly and aggressively even when they are discovered early. An important goal for oncologists is to be able to determine at the time of diagnosis which cancers have a bad prognosis. This has two major benefits. First, women with aggressive cancers could then get appropriate aggressive treatment. Second, women whose cancers do not fit that category would not be subject to six months or more of chemotherapy. A number of very promising areas of research are those that are identifying the biological characteristics of breast cancers that make them either good or bad risks.

Some breast cancers require a supply of the female hormone estrogen to grow. For women with this type of cancer, blocking the estrogen supply with hormones or drugs can stop or slow the tumor's growth. The most common anti-estrogen drug is tamoxifen, which has now become the most common form of adjuvant therapy for breast cancer. Tamoxifen also has the advantage of causing few of the side effects associated with chemotherapy.

How long adjuvant therapy lasts will vary, but it usually takes about six months. Four drugs are commonly used: Cytoxan (C), Methotrexate (M), Flourouracil (F), and Adriamycin (A). Three of these drugs are usually given in combination, sometimes with hormonal treatments.

Despite our best efforts, some breast cancers do recur or are diagnosed after they have already metastasized to another place in the body. Then the goals of treatment become to control the disease, prolong survival, and minimize symptoms, allowing the patient to live as normally as possible. Approximately 50 percent to 60 percent of metastatic breast cancers respond to treatment.

The drugs most commonly used are the same ones listed above. Some drugs can be taken indefinitely, although others are limited by their toxicity to normal tissues. Adriamycin, for example, will damage the heart at certain dose levels.

Another problem limiting the effectiveness of drug therapy is resistance. Many tumors eventually outsmart the drugs by developing resistance to their mechanism for killing cancer cells. Researchers at major centers around the country are working to develop ways of overcoming this problem, but drug resistance remains a serious obstacle to successful treatment of metastatic disease.

There has been considerable interest during the last few years in bone marrow transplants for advanced breast cancer. Bone marrow transplantation has become a useful form of therapy for certain other cancers, such as leukemias and lymphomas. This created the hope that it would cure some advanced solid tumors as well. The theory is that one huge dose of anticancer therapy would be sufficient to destroy all existing cancer cells. The only way to find out if that is true is to do a clinical trial comparing bone marrow transplants with other forms of therapy. This trial would allow researchers to compare the length of survival of the patients receiving each type of treatment and to study some important issues related to quality of life.

One such major trial is currently under way in Philadelphia, Pennsylvania, where four medical centers are cooperating with a major insurer to study bone marrow transplants in women with advanced breast cancer. This and other studies like it will yield important information about the value of this treatment approach.

The real hope for progress in breast cancer lies in understanding why these cancers occur and in developing ways to break the chain of events that leads to malignancy.

Ovarian Cancer

Compared to breast cancer, most women know very little about *ovarian cancer*, yet it is far from rare. Each year about twenty-two thousand

American women will learn that they have this disease. It is the fourth leading cancer killer of women in this country, accounting for more than thirteen thousand deaths a year.

The causes of ovarian cancer are poorly understood. The ovaries lie deep within the pelvis. During a woman's reproductive life, they release eggs, or ova, on a monthly basis during ovulation. The ovary is involved in major hormonal cycles. In addition, with every ovulation, the surface of the ovary tears as the egg is pushed out into the Fallopian tube and carried to the uterus. Many researchers believe that continuous ovulation eventually leads to an error in the repair process and to the development of abnormal or cancerous cells. That could explain, in part, why women who interrupt the ovulatory cycle through pregnancy, breastfeeding, or oral contraceptives have lower rates of ovarian cancer. Researchers are still searching for other genetic or environmental factors that increase a woman's risk of getting ovarian cancer.

The most important known risk factor for ovarian cancer is getting older. Most ovarian cancers occur in women older than age sixty. Unfortunately, many women stop seeing their gynecologists on a regular basis after they reach menopause. That is a mistake—the need for regular pelvic examinations continues throughout a woman's life. Women who have never had children or who had difficulty conceiving are also at increased risk of ovarian cancer. There has been a good deal of media publicity about familial ovarian cancers—those that occur in one or more family members. However, these account for less than 10 percent of all ovarian cancers. If one or more of your close relatives—a grandmother, mother, sister, or aunt—had this cancer, you should be sure that you have frequent checkups and that you have made your doctor aware of your family history.

There are some gynecologic oncologists who advocate removing the ovaries of women with strong family histories of ovarian cancer. In addition to their risk, many of these women have high levels of fear and anxiety about the possibility of developing ovarian cancer. This approach, however, involves major surgery, which in itself carries a small but real risk. In addition, those with multiple relatives with ovarian cancer involve only one-half of 1 percent of all ovarian cancers. Moreover, for women with a documented genetic risk of ovarian cancer, removing the ovaries does not guarantee protection. A small percentage of women who undergo the preventive surgery still go on to develop cancer in the pelvic cavity.

There is no test for ovarian cancer that is equivalent to mammography for breast cancer or to the Pap test for cervical cancer (the Pap test rarely detects ovarian cancer). Right now, the only way to detect this type of cancer is by having a thorough pelvic examination. In high-risk women, a test for a blood marker called CA125 is sometimes done. Elevated levels of CA125 can be an indication of ovarian cancer. The test is not accurate or specific enough to be used as a screening test for all women, however. If an abnormality is suspected, the physician may order a special procedure called a *transvaginal ultrasound,* for diagnostic purposes.

The symptoms of ovarian cancer are nonspecific. They include a persistent bloated feeling, back pain, pelvic pressure, or digestive disturbances. These are, of course, the symptoms of many other conditions as well, but any woman who experiences one or more of these symptoms should see a doctor and insist on a pelvic examination. The difficulty inherent in detecting ovarian cancer leads to a low survival rate, since 70 percent to 80 percent of these cancers are found in an advanced state. Despite some real progress, ovarian cancer remains difficult to diagnose early and treat successfully.

As with most cancers, the treatment for ovarian cancer depends largely on the extent of the disease. When a cancer is diagnosed, the patient goes through a process called "staging" to determine how large the tumor is and whether it has spread. *Stage I* ovarian cancers are those that have not spread beyond the ovary. These account for only about 25 percent of all ovarian cancers and are generally found on routine examinations. *Stage II* cancers involve both ovaries or extend to the pelvic area. *Stage III and IV* tumors have spread more distantly to other parts of the body.

Staging is done by surgical exploration of the pelvic area. It is very important that the staging be accurate. Women who are not correctly staged often do not receive adequate treatment for their disease. Stage I and II tumors are highly curable when they are treated correctly.

Surgery is the primary treatment for ovarian cancer. The goal is to remove all the cancer, but often this is not possible. Roughly two-thirds of all ovarian cancer patients have advanced disease at the time of diagnosis.

Most women with ovarian cancer require some form of follow-up treatment after surgery. This almost always involves chemotherapy or, less commonly, radiation therapy as well. In recent years, advances in the chemotherapy itself and in the way the drugs are delivered have improved the results of treatment. The use of platinum-based drugs has greatly increased the percentage of women who respond to chemotherapy.

One of the great frustrations of cancer treatment is that patients often respond very well to chemotherapy at the beginning. At some point, however, the drugs become ineffective, so the disease progresses. Frequently these patients do not respond well to other drug treatments. This drug resistance occurs when cancer cells change a key characteristic that allows them to escape the lethal effects of chemotherapy.

Ovarian cancers have a strong tendency to become drug resistant. Researchers at major cancer centers are focusing their efforts on understanding and circumventing the mechanisms that allow ovarian cancer cells to improve their defenses against drugs. Various clinical trials are being conducted to test agents designed to make these cells more sensitive to chemotherapy.

Another promising therapy for ovarian cancer is the drug taxol. Derived from the Western yew tree, taxol has attracted a great deal of attention from the media and from patients and their physicians because it has produced a consistently good response rate in women with advanced ovarian cancer. Until recently, taxol has been very difficult to obtain and has been in very short supply. This has changed because researchers have learned how to use the branches of the tree as well as the bark. Taxol is now widely available for patients with ovarian cancer and other tumors as well.

Taxol works differently from many other cancer drugs. To kill cancer cells, taxol interferes with the cell's ability to organize its genetic material, so the cancer cell cannot multiply and, instead, it dies. Numerous clinical trials now under way are using taxol for treating ovarian and other cancers. To date, these trials seem promising.

Treatment for ovarian cancer is complex and difficult. Patients often have numerous symptoms that require attention. Women with this cancer should definitely be treated in a cancer center with a multidisciplinary team and an experienced gynecologic oncologist. Properly treated, even women with advanced disease often survive for long periods of time and maintain a good quality of life.

In the future, we can expect to see improved methods of screening for ovarian cancer that will allow doctors to find it at an earlier stage. These methods will result from a better understanding of what makes cancer cells different from normal cells and from the ability to identify the products of abnormal cells. Researchers will continue to dedicate their efforts to the difficulties inherent in finding new agents that are effective against ovarian cancer and that can overcome the problem of drug resistance.

Uterine Cancer

Endometrial cancer, cancer of the lining of the uterus, or endometrium, is the most common gynecologic cancer in the United States and is one of the six leading causes of cancer deaths in women. During the first half of the twentieth century, cancer of the uterine cervix was three times more common than was endometrial cancer or other cancers in the body of the uterus, but this trend has been reversed. According to the American Cancer Society, in 1992 there were thirty-two thousand new cases of endometrial cancer and other noncervical cancers of the uterus.

Three-quarters of all endometrial cancers occur in women older than fifty, with the peak incidence occurring between ages fifty-eight and sixty. Overweight women with large body frames have a significantly higher rate of uterine cancer. Women who have diabetes and hypertension have increased rates of this cancer as well. As with most cancers, however, many women without known risk factors develop uterine cancer.

Uterine cancers are known to be hormone dependent. Women who have constant stimulation from estrogen with low levels of progesterone are at very high risk for endometrial cancer. For this reason, infertility and menstrual disorders, especially heavy bleeding at menopause, are risk factors.

The only symptom of endometrial cancer is abnormal bleeding or discharge. In postmenopausal women, abnormal bleeding indicates cancer about one-third of the time. In premenopausal women and those about to undergo menopause, a much smaller percentage of women with abnormal bleeding are found to have cancer.

Too many women stop seeing their gynecologists after they pass the childbearing age. It is just as important for a woman whose family is complete to see her doctor as it is for younger women. It is equally important to make sure that abnormal bleeding is evaluated. Pap smears, which are highly accurate in diagnosing cervical cancer, have only a 50 percent accuracy rate in diagnosing endometrial cancer. The best way to obtain an accurate diagnosis of this cancer is to take samples of the uterine tissue for biopsy, a procedure known as dilation and curettage (D and C).

Once a woman's cancer is diagnosed, she has a series of tests to determine the extent of the cancer. These include ultrasound, magnetic resonance imaging (MRI), and examinations of the urinary and lower gastrointestinal tracts. When these studies are complete, the cancer is staged, with stage I being the earliest and stage IV the most advanced.

There are a number of approaches to treating endometrial cancer. This is particularly true for cancers that have not spread beyond the uterus itself—about 75 percent of all cases. The standard treatment remains hysterectomy, but in some cancer centers, physicians recommend additional radiation therapy, either before or after the surgery.

The survival rate for women with early endometrial cancer—Stages I and II—is very high. Since most cases of uterine cancer are discovered in these early stages, the cure rates for this disease are generally high. Women with more advanced disease have a lower survival rate but can benefit greatly from treatment involving radiation and surgery, often combined with hormone treatment or chemotherapy. Some studies have also shown that hormone treatment using progestine after surgery or radiation reduces the recurrence rate for uterine cancer.

Cancer researchers are now working to find tumor markers to screen women for endometrial cancer and to signal recurrence before women have symptoms. Researchers are also trying to identify factors that put some patients at great risk for recurrence even when their disease appears to be in its early stages.

Cervical Cancer

Cancer of the uterine cervix is now the fifth most common cancer in American women, after cancer of the lung, breast, colon and rectum, and uterine lining. The American Cancer Society estimates that each year there are 13,500 cases of invasive *cervical cancer* and 4,400 deaths from this disease. There are also more than 55,000 cases of what is known as *carcinoma in situ of the cervix.*

The distinction made between invasive cervical cancer and carcinoma in situ of the cervix results from the widespread use of the Pap test to screen for cervical cancer. A Pap smear can often detect cells that have become abnormal before they have spread into adjacent areas. This condition is known as cancer *in situ,* meaning *in place.* These very early cancers or even precancerous abnormalities can be treated easily and almost 100 percent successfully.

Risk Factors

Low-income and minority women, both urban and rural, have much higher-than-average rates of cervical cancer. African American women, for example, are three times more likely to develop this cancer and twice as likely to die of it as are white women, according to National Cancer Institute studies. Latina women also are at increased risk, but women of Jewish and European origin have lower rates.

Women who begin having sexual intercourse at a young age, women who have multiple sexual partners, and women who have numerous pregnancies have the greatest incidence of cervical cancer. Women who have never been pregnant or who are sexually inactive seldom get this disease. Some researchers believe that male circumcision helps to protect women against cervical cancer, but studies done throughout the world have not fully supported this theory.

Although causes of cervical cancer are not yet known, a great deal of attention has focused on the human papilloma virus (HPV). This virus is spread by sexual contact. In populations in which a large percentage of people are infected with HPV, the incidence of cervical cancer is high. Researchers also find that a high percentage of women with cervical cancer are infected by the papilloma virus, as are a high percentage of their sexual partners.

Detection and Treatment

The Pap test is the ideal way to detect cervical cancer early. This exam is simple, inexpensive, and safe. It finds cancers before they become life-threatening, when they do not require extensive treatment. The existence of the Pap test makes it unnecessary for any woman to die of cervical cancer, yet 4,500 women in this country die from it every year.

Every woman who is sexually active or has reached age twenty-one should get regular Pap tests. Unfortunately, there has been some disagreement among the medical profession as to how often these tests are necessary. We recommend that women have three consecutive annual Pap tests. If those tests are all normal, then a woman can wait up to three years before getting another one. Women who are at high risk, however, should make an annual Pap smear an essential part of their regular health care.

Not every abnormal Pap smear indicates malignancy. Many abnormal smears result from infections or from precancerous lesions. Some of these conditions will heal by themselves or with drug treatment. Others that are precancerous require a procedure called a colposcopy to examine and biopsy the abnormal area. In most cases, these small precancerous areas, known as dysplasia, can be removed completely during the biopsy and do not require further treatment. Larger lesions are usually removed through a surgical procedure called conization.

The treatment for carcinoma in situ of the cervix depends largely on the patient's age and whether or not she wants to have more children. Older patients and those who are finished having children are best treated with hysterectomy. Women who do want children are treated more conservatively with laser surgery, cryosurgery, or conization.

In cases of invasive cervical cancer, the patient needs to have a series of tests to determine the extent of the disease. This staging process is essential to deciding on the correct treatment approach. The tests may include computerized axial tomography (CAT) scans, ultrasound examinations, MRI scans, or surgery. Cervical cancers are also staged as I to IV, with Stage I being the least extensive and Stage IV the most widespread. Stage I and II cervical cancers have very high cure rates, as do these stages of endometrial cancer.

Patients with early cervical cancer are treated with either surgery or radiation therapy designed to cure the disease. Radiation therapy and surgery have comparable cure rates. The choice is often based on the kinds of side effects that each treatment causes. Younger women often prefer surgery, which can preserve their ovaries and may not affect sexual function. For older or less sexually active women, radiation is often the treatment of choice.

Patients with more advanced disease are treated with radiation therapy alone. Chemotherapy has not proved useful in treating women with cervical cancer, although researchers are continuing to do trials to find effective drug combinations for advanced disease.

About the Author

Dr. Robert C. Young is president of Fox Chase Cancer Center, Philadelphia, one of twenty-eight National Cancer Institute–designated comprehensive can-

cer centers. *Internationally known for his work in the treatment of lymphoma and ovarian cancer, he is a past president of the American Society of Clinical Oncology (ASCO), one of the world's largest oncology societies.*

Dr. Young came to Fox Chase in 1988 from the National Cancer Institute (NCI), where he was associate director of the center and the community oncology program. Previously he served as chief of NCI's medicine branch for fourteen years.

Dr. Young is active in numerous professional societies and currently serves as the chair of the strategic planning committee of ASCO. He also chairs the subcommittee on Hodgkin's disease and lymphoma of the American Joint Committee on Cancer and is a member of the board of directors of the National Coalition for Cancer Research.

Dr. Young received his B. Sc. degree in zoology from Ohio State University and his M.D. from Cornell University Medical College. Following his internship at New York Hospital, he completed his residency at NCI and Yale–New Haven Medical Center.

QUESTIONS FOR THE DOCTOR

Q: **I have heard many stories of women who have been told by their doctors that they do not have any suspicious lumps in their breasts or have been told that their mammograms are normal; yet, they have pursued the issue and have found that, in fact, they do have breast cancer. What is your advice to women in this situation?**

A: There is a great deal to be said for using your judgment and following your instinct. If you believe deep down that you have a breast mass, or if you notice what appears to be a significant change in your breast tissue, you should not hesitate to seek a second opinion. I do not know of a physician who should be insulted by a person searching out additional help for his or her health care. Most important in this arrangement between a physician and a patient is keeping the patient healthy. Patients play a very important part. It is clear that the current techniques to evaluate breast cancer are far from perfect, and it is essential that people play a critical role in their own care.

To that end I would strongly suggest that all women do a monthly breast self-examination. In addition, men should periodically check to see if they have any abnormal lumps or growth in their breast tissue. Although breast cancer occurs rarely in men, it does occur and is a concern.

Q: *I have been told I have* fibrocystic breast disease. *Am I at greater risk for breast cancer?*

A: That is a difficult question to answer. Fibrocystic breast disease is actually not a disease but a predisposition to have lumpy breasts. In the past, numerous studies indicated that you are at greater risk for breast cancer if you have this disease. Recently, however, physicians realized that they were finding greater numbers of cases of breast cancer in women with fibrocystic breast disease because these women's cases were followed more closely and they had more routine biopsies. Fifty percent of women have fibrocystic breasts. In fact, many doctors now hesitate to call this a disease because it occurs so often. Certainly, the vast majority of these women do not develop breast cancer. The difficulty is that fibrocystic breasts are far more difficult to examine because you or your doctor may feel nodularities in certain areas, which can be confused with lumps. That is why it is important for you to be taught by your physician how to do a proper breast exam. The major problem with fibrocystic breast disease is that it can be quite painful. Physicians have found that reducing caffeine and other similar products can actually help with the pain.

Q: *Are nipples part of the breast tissue and, if they are, can they become cancerous?*

A: Certainly, nipples can become cancerous; they are a part of the breast. The disease that affects the nipple the most is Paget's disease. It is associated with 1 percent to 3 percent of breast cancers and it seems to affect women in their fifties the most. Although the condition occurs in men, it is quite rare. The disease actually is started in the ducts underneath the nipple. Most patients who have the problem have a dry, scaly, eczematous lesion of the nipple. The nipple is tender and there may also be a discharge. If a woman has a discharge from her nipple, and she is not in the late stages of pregnancy or she is not breastfeeding, she should consult her doctor.

Q: *I have noticed abnormal vaginal bleeding for the past four months. After my period is over, it seems to start again about ten days later. Is there anything that I should worry about?*

A: Yes, you should see your gynecologist as soon as possible. Abnormal uterine bleeding can be a sign of many things, but one of the concerns is cancer, and, certainly, the bleeding should be evaluated.

3

Children's Immunizations, Diet, and Behavior

Rosemary Casey, M.D.

All parents who have experienced the joy of holding their newborn infant in their arms know the incredible happiness this child has brought into their lives. They marvel at each new developmental milestone, and they strive to meet every need of this new human being. They know immediately that, along with great joy, parenthood brings a burden of responsibility for the well-being of their baby. Most parents worry more about the health of their children than they do about their own health. They have many questions and concerns about their infants and children because nothing in their past experience really prepared them completely for the challenges of parenthood. This chapter cannot cover every question, but it focuses on some basic areas in pediatric primary care: immunizations, nutrition and cholesterol, and common behavioral problems. This basic information provides a foundation for further discussion with your pediatrician about your child's individual needs.

Immunizations

Immunizations play a critical role in maintaining the well-being of children. Over the last three years, outbreaks of measles in Los Angeles, Dallas, Chicago, New York, and Philadelphia, as well as increases in whooping cough and mumps elsewhere in the United States, indicate that we are failing to give every child one of the most basic components of good health care. Though the urban preschool child is at greatest risk for failing to be immunized, national statistics indicate that immunization rates among U.S. preschool children are disappointingly low, and they appear to be falling steadily. Informed parents can be the best advocates for their children. You will be more likely to keep your child's shots up to date if you know the recommended immunization schedule.

It is a good idea to keep a record of your child's shots with you at all times. If you receive a call that your child has been injured at camp or if your child is injured while your family is away on vacation, you will then be able to tell the treating physician which tetanus shots, for example, your child has received. It is also important to have the immunization record with you whenever you are visiting your child's physician. Even though the visit may be for a mild cold or a minor cut, your child can receive the necessary immunizations during this office visit. Very often physicians do not see the immunization record at these times and they fail to immunize the child. These are "missed opportunities" that contribute to the low immunization rates in the United States.

The schedule of vaccinations recommended for all children by the American Academy of Pediatrics appears in Table 3–1. Most experts agree that these are the appropriate ages to receive these immunizations, but as the chart shows, alternative timing is recommended by some experts. Note that the combined diptheria, tetanus, and pertussis vaccine (DTP) and the polio vaccine can be given at fifteen months or at eighteen months. Some physicians recommend that the last immunization with the combined measles, mumps, and rubella vaccine (MMR) be given later than ages four to six years and suggest waiting until the child enters middle school or junior high school.

Both the haemophilus b conjugate vaccine (HIB), a vaccine to fight a common cause of ear infections and meningitis, and the hepatitis B vaccine (HB) can be given at different intervals. Discuss these variations with your physician to find out which one he or she recommends; then you can make a note on your child's immunization record as a reminder about which schedule you will be using. You will also want to know if your child will be receiving several vaccines at once or if your physician recommends giving them one at a time. The latter method will mean that you will have to schedule more office visits.

These guidelines are currently up-to-date, but they can change as new research is reported. All pediatricians who are Fellows of the American Academy of Pediatrics receive updated schedules as new information

TABLE 3-1
The American Academy of Pediatrics Schedule of Recommended Vaccinations

Vaccine	Birth	1 Mo.	2 Mos.	4 Mos.	6 Mos.	12 Mos.	15 Mos.	18 Mos.	4–6 Yrs.[c]
DTP			√	√	√		√	[or √]	√
Polio			√	√			√	[or √]	√
MMR						[√ or]	√	√[b]	
HIB									
4-dose option			√	√	√		√		
3-dose option			√	√		√			

	1–2 Mos.		6–18 Mos.	
HB				
Option 1	√[a]		√[a]	
Option 2	√[a]	√[a]	√[a]	

[a]Can be given with DTP, polio, MMR, or HIB.
[b]Many experts recommend that this dose of MMR vaccine be given at entry to middle school or junior high school.
[c]Before school entry.
Source: U.S. Department of Health and Human Services, Public Health Service, *Diptheria, Tetanus, and Pertussis: What You Need to Know*. Atlanta: Centers for Disease Control, 1991.

on immunizations becomes available. You should not be surprised, however, if your doctor's recommendations change before your child receives the full complement of vaccinations or if the schedule for a younger child is different from that of an older child.

Diphtheria, Tetanus, Pertussis (DTP)

The DTP vaccine is one shot against three diseases. *Diphtheria* is a very serious disease that can cause extreme difficulty in breathing, paralysis, or heart failure. Fortunately, only a few cases of diphtheria are reported in the United States each year because most people have had immunizations against it. *Tetanus* (lockjaw) makes a person unable to open his or her mouth to swallow because of severe muscle spasms; it occurs after a cut or wound lets the germ into the body. *Pertussis* (whooping cough) causes severe spells of coughing or choking that make it hard to eat, drink, or breathe. It is most dangerous for those infants who are less than twelve months old. As many as sixteen out of one hundred babies with pertussis get pneumonia, and two out of one hundred may have seizures or convulsions. About one out of every two hundred babies with pertussis dies of it. Every year as many as forty-two hundred cases of pertussis are reported in the United States, and many cases are not diagnosed or reported.

There are some side effects associated with the DTP vaccine. Most children have little or no problem from the DTP shot, although a slight fever or soreness and swelling where the shot was given are relatively common. A few children (fewer than one out of one hundred) will cry excessively for three or more hours. The cry may be unusually high-pitched. The DTP immunization may cause some children to run a high temperature, sometimes greater than 105 degrees. In rare cases (less than one out of fifteen hundred times), a child may have a seizure or convulsions (usually from a high fever), or a child may become blue or pale and limp, a condition called shock or collapse. Despite these reactions, medical experts believe that most children should receive the DTP immunization.

Many parents become alarmed or confused by news stories about children who have had bad reactions to a particular vaccine. For example, very rarely, permanent brain damage has been reported after a child received a DTP shot, but most experts agree that the DTP vaccine has not been shown to be the cause of the brain damage. Children who show some sign of a brain problem, such as uncontrolled seizures or convulsions, should not be given the DTP vaccine.

A child who has experienced adverse reactions to the initial injection should not receive any more in the series of DTP immunizations. For example, a doctor would not give a DTP shot to a child who had a severe allergic reaction, marked by mouth or throat swelling, within a few hours of receiving a previous DTP shot. Children with such adverse reactions can receive combined diptheria and tetanus (DT) vaccine instead. Your physician knows the specific situations in which to delay or withhold a DTP shot. You should be sure to get clear instructions from your doctor about the kinds of reactions to watch for after your child has received his or her vaccination. You need to be alert to the reactions that indicate a serious problem so that neither you nor the child will be unduly upset about the common and temporary reactions. The important point is that the number of children who have a problem after receiving the DTP vaccine is very small. It is crucial to remember that children, especially infants, who get diptheria, tetanus, or pertussis can become very ill and may die.

Polio

Polio is a very dangerous disease that causes severe muscle pain and paralysis, the inability to move the arms, legs, or the muscle that enables people to breathe. Many parents remember the 1952 epidemic, when more than twenty thousand people were paralyzed by polio. Although there are few cases of polio in the United States now, there are still thousands of cases of polio each year in other countries. Therefore, it is important to protect children with vaccines so that they cannot get polio if the virus is carried into the United States from another country.

What are the risks of the various polio vaccines? Live oral polio vaccine (OPV) is given as drops in the mouth: The polio virus is still alive but has been made very weak. Very rarely, once every 1.5 million doses, OPV causes polio in the person who gets the drops or in people who are in close contact with the person who gets the vaccine. For instance, stool in diapers can be a source of spread. This is a particular risk for adults who have never received polio vaccine; these adults should be vaccinated with inactivated polio vaccine before or at the same time as the child.

Inactivated polio vaccine (IPV) is given as a shot, and the polio virus used in the shot has been killed. The injection can cause a little soreness or redness where the vaccine enters the body. Instead of OPV, IPV is given to a child who has a condition, such as cancer, leukemia, or AIDS, that makes it hard to fight infections. If an adult in the child's household has one of these conditions, doctors usually give IPV rather than OPV.

Experts agree that the benefits of receiving the polio vaccines outweigh the risks. There are some children, however, who may need to delay receiving the polio vaccine or who should not receive it at all.

Measles, Mumps, and Rubella (MMR)

The MMR vaccine, like the DTP vaccine, is one injection against three diseases. *Measles* is a common but serious disease that causes high fever, cough, and a rash and lasts for one to two weeks. It can also cause an infection of the brain that leads to convulsions, hearing loss, and mental retardation. Babies and adults who catch measles are much sicker and are more likely to die than are schoolage children who contract the disease. During the 1990 measles epidemic, twenty-five thousand cases of the disease and more than sixty deaths attributed to it were reported.

Mumps causes fever, headache, and swollen, painful glands under the jaw. It, too, can be a serious disease. Mumps sometimes causes *meningitis* (an inflammation of the lining of the brain), which can paralyze or kill. About one person in every ten who get mumps also gets meningitis.

Rubella, or German measles, usually causes a mild disease with fever, swollen glands, and a rash. However, rubella is very dangerous to the unborn baby of a pregnant woman who has not been protected against rubella (about one out of every ten women in the United States).

Most people who get the MMR vaccine will not have a problem. About five children out of one hundred will get a rash one or two weeks after receiving the measles vaccine, and some children have fever with the rash. Rarely (in one out of one hundred patients), the rubella vaccine will cause pain or stiffness in the joints that may last up to three days.

Overall, the benefits of receiving the MMR vaccine outweigh the risks. Your physician knows that certain children should delay receiving an MMR injection or should not receive it at all. For example, a child with cancer, leukemia, AIDS, or any condition that impairs the ability to fight infection would not normally receive an MMR vaccination. A child with a severe allergic reaction to eggs might require special consideration before receiving a measles vaccine. The MMR vaccine, in part, is grown in an egg medium and some people have reactions to this.

Haemophilus Influenza B (HIB)

Haemophilus influenza type B is a germ that causes severe infections in one out of every two hundred children younger than age five in the United States. To prevent this disease, the HIB vaccine is commonly used. The bacteria that the HIB vaccine protect against cause over half of all cases of bacterial meningitis. About 5 percent of children who develop *haemophilus B meningitis* die, regardless of the treatment they receive. Those who survive often have permanent disabilities, including mental retardation and hearing loss. Haemophilus influenza type B also causes *epiglottiditis,* an infection of the small flap at the back of the throat that prevents food from going down the windpipe. If not treated immediately, the swelling can block the windpipe and cause death. In addition, haemophilus influenza type B can cause serious infections of the joints, bones, and skin tissues.

Most children who receive the HIB vaccine will not have any adverse reaction. HIB vaccines may cause fever, redness, and swelling where the shot is given.

Experts agree that all children should be immunized against haemophilus influenza type B. This vaccine has recently been proven to be effective in very young infants (age two months), and so parents of all children less than age five should take the opportunity to immunize their young children against haemophilus influenza type B.

Hepatitus B (HB)

Hepatitis B vaccine is now frequently given to prevent *hepatitis B* infection, which ranges from a mild viral illness with nausea, loss of appetite, and fatigue to a very serious, sometimes fatal, hepatitis (or liver infection). Children often have milder symptoms than do adults, but those people who have hepatitis B as children are at risk to be "chronic carriers" of the virus. Chronic carriers, especially those infected at a young age, are at increased risk of developing cirrhosis and liver cancer. An estimated one million Americans are chronic carriers of hepatitus B. Five thousand people die each year in the United States from complications of hepatitis B infection; therefore, the American Academy of Pediatrics Committee on Infectious Diseases has recommended that all newborns receive the HB vaccine, which has been proven to be very safe. The hepatitis B virus is spread through contact with blood and through sexual activity. Teenagers and young adults are at particular risk and should be vaccinated. The goal is to achieve universal immunization of all children, but this is a recommendation, not a requirement. You should discuss this recommendation with your child's physician.

New Recommendations

DTaP is the new acellular pertussis vaccine that is made from only a few parts of the pertussis cell. It is then combined with diphtheria and tetanus vaccines. (The DTP vaccine is made from killed whole pertussis cells.) Compared with the DTP vaccine, the DTaP injections cause less fever and soreness where the shot is given. However, until further testing shows that the DTaP vaccine is safe and effective for infants, it can be given only to children fifteen to eighteen months old and four to six years old.

Nutrition and Cholesterol

Parents realize that their baby's nutritional needs during the rapid-growth period of infancy are greater than at any other time in life. The baby's birth weight triples during the first year. Human milk is the ideal food for human infants because of its nutritional composition. It also contains substances that provide additional immunity against infection, and it is least likely to cause allergic reactions; therefore, most pediatricians urge mothers to breastfeed. Many factors affect this individual decision, however, and an expectant mother should weigh the various considerations and make a decision about breastfeeding before her infant is born.

Infant formula is a nutritious alternative to human milk. It is important that you do not feel guilty if you decide that bottle feeding is the best way for you to feed your infant. You can often combine breastfeeding and bottle feeding during the infant's first six months.

Infants should receive breast milk or formula, without any other foods, from birth to age four months. Young infants do not have the muscle control in their tongues and mouths to handle solids before four months. Between four and six months, babies often seem persistently hungry. They also need additional iron, which is provided in iron-fortified cereal. When you begin to feed your baby solid foods, your pediatrician will usually recommend that you start with rice cereal, the least allergenic food. You may gradually add other cereals, fruits, and vegetables, and then pureed meats between six and twelve months of age.

Shortly after the baby's first birthday, parents often become concerned by the decline in their toddler's appetite. Mealtimes used to be fun, but they can now become real battles. It is important to remember that your child's growth rate has slowed down, and he or she does not require as much food. You should offer foods from the four basic nutrition groups: (1) meat, fish, poultry, and eggs; (2) dairy products; (3) fruits and vegetables; and (4) cereal, grains, potatoes, and pasta. If the child refuses to finish a meal or to eat some foods, however, don't fight about it. If you refuse to allow your children to fill up on empty-calorie foods such as cookies or sweets between meals, their caloric needs will usually be met over several days from their regular diets, which should include *nutritious* snack foods.

Cholesterol

Most parents are aware that elevated cholesterol levels are related to heart and blood vessel disease in adulthood. The process of atherosclerosis (a buildup of fatty deposits in the walls of blood vessels that causes their diameter to narrow) begins in childhood. Unfortunately, American children have higher blood cholesterol levels and higher intakes of saturated fatty acids and cholesterol than do children in other countries.

Some parents try to restrict fat and cholesterol in young infants and toddlers. This is a dangerous practice. The American Academy of Pediatrics has made specific recommendations for children in its "National Cholesterol Education Program Report of the Expert Panel on Blood Cholesterol Levels in Children and Adolescents." These recommendations, however, are not intended for infants from birth to two years of age, whose fast growth requires a higher percentage of calories from fat. Two- and three-year-old toddlers may safely make the transition to the recommended eating pattern as they begin to eat with the family.

In brief, the general advice of the expert panel is that children can achieve adequate nutrition by eating a wide variety of foods. The daily intake of calories for energy should be sufficient to support growth and development and to reach or maintain desirable body weight. Recommendations for the daily maximum number of calories change with the child's age, of course, but at every age there are specific guidelines for controlling the proportion of fat in the diet. An average of no more than 30 percent of total daily calories should come from fat. Less than 10 percent of total daily calories should come from saturated fatty acid. The daily diet of children and adolescents should have less than 30 milligrams of cholesterol.

Each of the recommendations given above is intended as an average over a period of several days rather than an absolute measure for every single day. To achieve this nutritional goal, the panel recommends that families select, prepare, and consume foods low in saturated fatty acids, total fat, and cholesterol. Choosing a variety of foods ensures that everyone in the family will consume adequate amounts of carbohydrates, protein, and other nutrients. Like adults, children should consume only enough calories to maintain desirable weight. This eating pattern supports normal growth and development; it provides enough total energy, and meets or exceeds the Recommended Dietary Allowances (RDA) for all nutrients for children and adolescents, including iron and calcium.

Of course it is always easier to state a recommendation than to follow it. The following suggestions will help you reduce saturated fats during food preparation:

- Prepare meats, chicken, and fish by baking, broiling, roasting; stew meats ahead of time and skim accumulated fat from the surface.
- When cooking foods such as eggs, French toast, and pancakes, brush the pan with vegetable oil just to coat it, or use a nonstick pan.

- Use low-fat or skim milk in place of whole milk in recipes; use low-fat or nonfat yogurt in place of regular yogurt or sour cream.
- Reduce the number of egg yolks used in recipes or use egg substitutes for some or all of the eggs required in recipes.
- Do not spread bread with margarine, butter, or high-fat dressings when making sandwiches.
- Do not add fatty sauces to vegetables; try flavoring vegetables with lemon juice, herbs, or yogurt-based sauces.

Many pediatric practices have adopted routine cholesterol testing despite a lack of evidence that such screening programs can be effectively included in routine well-child care. The National Cholesterol Education Panel and the American Academy of Pediatrics Committee on Nutrition recommend limited cholesterol testing. This means that you should have your child's cholesterol checked only if

- he or she is more than two years old *and*
- someone in your family has had a high cholesterol level (over 240 mg/dl) or a high level of lipids, *or*
- someone in your family has had a heart attack or myocardial infarction before age fifty-five.

Your child's screening cholesterol will be considered abnormal if it is greater than 175 mg/dl (the 75th percentile). Children with borderline and elevated screening values need to have fasting lipid panels (total cholesterol, triglycerides, high-density lipoprotein cholesterol) before they are labeled as "hypercholesterolemic." Families of children with elevated cholesterol are advised to have several visits with a dietician to review family eating patterns and nutritious, low-cholesterol, low saturated-fat diets.

Good Eating Habits

Realize that your young child needs quite a bit of food to grow and develop properly and that he or she cannot get adequate nutrition in just three meals a day. You should plan for regular and healthy between-meal snacks; your child's appetite will vary from time to time and you will need some flexibility in responding to the changes. Refer to the nutrition chapter in this book for planning family meals as well as snacks. The same guidelines for nutritious meals apply to snacks. Children should not be routinely snacking on the high-fat, high-sugar foods that you avoid giving them in regular meals. Fruits, small sandwiches, vegetables, and good cereals with low-fat milk all make better snacks than candy, greasy chips, cakes, or cookies. With so many health-conscious convenience foods available, parents do not have to deprive children of enjoyable foods or spend any time at all in preparing special snacks. Children are bombarded with advertisements and other messages about fast-food restaurants, snack foods, and empty-calorie cereals. When children who are just learning to talk already recognize corporate logos and characters associated with "kids" foods, parents understandably have difficulty in avoiding such products. If you allow the fast burgers and sugar-laden cereals to be only an occasional departure from balanced family meals, your child will be learning a health-promoting approach to food that will last a lifetime.

Behavioral Problems

There are many books outlining the major developmental milestones in the first two years of life. Although the developmental tasks are the same for all children, each child approaches the challenge with a unique combination of temperament, genetic and environmental influences, and parental expectations. This results in a broad range of normal development, and the majority of children achieve each developmental task successfully. Therefore, this section will focus on the more common behavioral problems of the toddler and older child, with particular emphasis on the normal limits and signs that intervention is necessary.

Separation Anxiety

Separation anxiety—worry or upset that occurs when the child is temporarily away from a parent or home—is an appropriate response for preschoolers. A toddler is struggling with independence; he or she might, for example, insist on walking alone or running some distance away from a parent but will become inconsolable if the parent is out of sight for even a brief time. By first grade, a child usually is comfortable in the world of his or her peers, away from parents for much of the day. Selma Fraiberg and other child-development experts think that some anxiety may be crucial to the child's development of a mature ego-structure and personality. Parents should not be overly protective or too quick to prevent the child from feeling anxious about an unpleasant experience.

Children who fail to learn how to handle such experiences can develop *separation anxiety disorder.*

The diagnosis of this disorder is inappropriate during the child's preschool years or during the first months of school attendance, however, when elevated anxiety is expected. If your older child seems unable to handle separation or describes persistent morbid fears or phobias of kidnapping, accidents, or dying, there is cause for concern. These children frequently have nightmares and difficulty falling asleep, particularly if they are away from home. Their anxiety can take the form of physical complaints, such as headache or stomachache, or it can show up as school avoidance. If your child seems to have a separation anxiety disorder, consult your doctor about the need for psychiatric evaluation and help.

Fears and Phobias

Young children have a variety of common fears, including fears of animals, darkness, and loud noises. Girls tend to be more fearful than boys, and the fears of both girls and boys seem to peak when they are three years old. School-age children may also fear ghosts, monsters, and certain animals, but their fears shift to more abstract concepts such as dying. Fear can be a healthy emotion—for instance, when there is real danger and it is helpful in preventing physical injury. Fear is unhealthy when it is excessive (exaggerates danger) or spreads into an area in which there is no danger, thus interfering with the child's normal activities. For the most part, children manage their fears pretty well. Young children who still think of their parents as having special powers to protect them can usually overcome small anxieties with parental reassurance. Older children overcome their fears by intellectualizing them or by playing through them by acting tough or reading monster and horror stories. Because most children succeed in handling their fears, phobias are rare. A *phobia* is a persistent, excessive fear of a specific object that results in a desire to avoid that object or situation. The usual fear of insects or darkness is not considered a phobia unless avoidance of the object is significantly stressful for the child and interferes with normal social functioning. Children with phobias usually know that they should not be afraid. They do not want to be afraid and may suffer from the consequences of their avoidance behaviors. These children usually recover quite well, but treatment by experienced psychiatrists or psychologists is needed.

Temper Tantrums

Parents commonly ask how to deal with the temper tantrums that occur in children between the ages of six months and six years and are most frequent between the ages of one and three years. Tantrums reflect a child's struggle to become more autonomous and are often caused by frustration at failing to master a developmental task. Your child's doctor will ask about the frequency and specific circumstances of the tantrums and your feelings or reactions to your child's behavior. It is normal for a parent to feel angry or frustrated, but parents who relate only negative comments (e.g., "she's always being evil") are having significant parent-child interaction problems. In general, parents should help the child regain self-control (this can be done by holding the younger child or calling a "cooling-off period" in a safe place for the older child). Discipline should include praise for the desired behavior as well as disapproval for the undesired behavior. If your child has temper tantrums that control the household or that are constant, this may indicate that you and your child have lost control. If this is the case, you should ask your child's doctor for some specific suggestions to make life easier for both you and your child.

Toilet Training

Successful toilet training cannot occur before a child develops bowel and bladder control. That control is determined mainly by maturation and generally occurs between ages one and three. However, problems with toilet training are also a classic example of the toddler's struggle for autonomy. The outcome of this struggle is largely determined by the child's temperament, the parents' attitudes, and the parent-child interaction. Toilet training is usually successful when parents adopt a relaxed, nonthreatening approach once the child is ready. T. Barry Brazelton refers to this as a "child-oriented approach to toilet training." In this method, parents are taught to wait until the child is physically and psychologically ready (approximately at age two). Once the "potty chair" is casually introduced, the child moves gradually from sitting down on it while fully dressed, to changing soiled diapers on it, and eventually to using the potty chair correctly. Whenever your child fails or resists going to the next step, you need to wait and reassure the child about having mastered the current stage. Focus on your child's achievement, and do not feel that the pressure is on you. Most children should have bowel and daytime bladder control by age three to three and a half. Nighttime bladder control should be achieved by age five or six.

About the Author

Dr. Rosemary Casey is a native Philadelphian who attended Immaculata College. She received her M.D. degree from Harvard Medical School in 1975. Following pediatric residency training at the Children's Hospital of Philadelphia, she pursued additional study in epidemiology, sociology, and research design as a Robert Wood Johnson Clinical Scholar at the University of Pennsylvania. Since then, Dr. Casey has continued her broad-based interests in the practice of pediatrics, clinical research, and the education of pediatric residents and medical students.

Dr. Casey is assistant professor of pediatrics at the University of Pennsylvania School of Medicine and director of the General Pediatric Faculty Practice at the Children's Hospital of Philadelphia. She currently serves as regional co-chair of the Ambulatory Pediatric Association.

QUESTIONS FOR THE DOCTOR

Q: *Can cigarette smoke hurt my child's asthma?*
A: There is no doubt that cigarette smoke can be an irritant to a child's airways. Studies have shown that it can make asthma worse. Perhaps more important, studies have also shown that cigarette smoke can cause lung cancer and dramatic changes in people who do not smoke but who passively inhale cigarette smoke. Remember, when you are smoking you are hurting your spouse, your children, and all of those around you.

Q: *What sort of things should I do to ensure that my house is safe for my baby?*
A: You can do a number of things to "child-proof" your home and some of them are very simple. First, make sure you have some syrup of ipecac on hand in case your child swallows a poison. If your child does swallow a poison, you must first call your doctor or the poison control center and identify the poison your child ingested. If you are told to give ipecac, it will help rid the stomach of the offending poison. Certain poisons, however, such as drain cleaner, should not be treated with ipecac. Second, make sure that all electrical outlets either have child-protective caps or are not accessible to your child.

Children are seen in emergency rooms every day with serious burns that are the result of electrical injuries. Third, make sure that you have locks on your cabinets and that you label potentially poisonous substances and move them far out of reach of your child. And do not underestimate your child. Children are natural explorers, and this can lead to trouble. Fourth, if your child is old enough to ride a bike, make sure that he or she wears a safety helmet. Head injuries are still far too common. When you are traveling in a car, be sure to place your child in a car seat if he or she is at a young age or buckle your child's seatbelt if he or she is older. A child can easily become a projectile in an automobile accident and may sustain severe head and facial trauma. Finally, make sure that there is no way that your child can get near open windows. Do not assume that screens are a protection against children falling out; they are meant to keep insects out of the house, not keep children inside. Talk with your pediatrician about specific things that worry you.

Q: *I have a three-year old and a one-month old. I feel that I am not giving either of them enough time. Do you think I'm a bad mother?*

A: Probably not. The mere fact that you are asking this question indicates that you are concerned about your children's well-being. You now have two children, which means you probably have at least four times the amount of work to do as when you had one child. Try to pay attention to both of your children and address their needs, but do not feel guilty.

Q: *My child has a bright red eye, and it has been causing him pain for two days. The day-care center won't allow him in because they say that he has "pink eye." What is pink eye?*

A: Most day-care centers and schools are very frightened of pink eye, and for good reason. In true cases of pink eye, or *conjunctivitis,* the infectious agent is easily transmitted from child to child. It takes only a few days of antibiotic treatment to heal pink eye. However, there are other things that mimic this condition, including allergic symptoms. Children who have allergies often get red eyes. Doctors can distinguish conjunctivitis from allergic red eyes because the former usually occurs in one eye, whereas allergies usually affect both. Once again, you need to see your doctor to determine the diagnosis. In some cases the doctor may have to order an eye culture to see if a bacteria is causing the problem.

Q: *My child is three years old and is not toilet trained. All my friends' children are toilet trained. I'm getting very upset. What should I do?*

A: The first thing to do is to check with your doctor to make sure that every other stage of your child's development is coming along nicely. There is a direct relationship between emotional and physical development and age of toilet training. It is not unusual for toddlers to have problems with toilet training. Some children are very quick, and others are not. Reward a successful potty effort, but be sure that you do not punish an unsuccessful effort. Make toilet time a time for the child to look forward to, not a time to fear punishment. But, most important, do not assume that you are doing something wrong; maybe the child is just not ready.

Q: *My child's breast bone seems to protrude much more than other children's. Should I be concerned?*
A: I have not examined your child so I would certainly say it is important that you take your child to a pediatrician for an exam. However, a common problem is *pectus excavatum,* in which the sternum tends to stick out in a pronounced fashion. Usually there is no cause for concern.

Q: *My twelve-year-old son is very embarrassed because he is developing breasts. I took a look at him at the pool the other day, and he is. I'm concerned. Could he have a problem?*
A: As many as one in five adolescent boys developes breast buds through the early stages of adolescence. These usually go away over time. Some boys may even develop a breast bud on one side and not on the other. You can reassure your son by explaining that this is a normal development and that he need not be afraid of future problems. You can do little to prevent other children from making fun of him, but if he understands what is going on, he may be able to handle teasing better.

Q: *When is the best age to talk to my children about sex?*
A: The answer, unfortunately, has changed over the past several years because of the prevalence of HIV. It is critical that you warn your child about the potential danger of unprotected sexual intercourse. Furthermore, it is very important that you teach your child about his or her own body. Set up an open line of communication. You may want to check your local library for help in finding age-appropriate material that will help you discuss these important matters. The problems of child abuse have been well documented, and it is very important that your children know that they can and should tell you if anyone does or says something inappropriate to them. They must not be afraid to come to you. Talking about these subjects with your chil-

dren may be very embarrassing for both parents and children and may seem premature for a young child, but in today's world there is no way to avoid it. Do not assume that your child's school is providing this education. It may be difficult to talk about these issues with your children, but they need to know that you are there to help them if a problem occurs.

Q: *My child complains of stomachaches and has missed at least fifteen days of school in the last six months. I have gone to see doctors, and they have said there is nothing wrong with my child's stomach. Do you think they are making a mistake and missing something?*

A: It is difficult to know without examining your child. One possibility is that the child is trying to avoid a difficult situation by pretending to be sick. Complaints of stomach pain are very typical of this avoidance behavior. You should explore the possibility that your child just does not want to go to school and is trying to avoid the real problem.

Q: *I took my child to the pediatrician the other day, and he was concerned that my child may have a hearing problem. He referred me to a hearing specialist, but my health insurance does not cover the referral and I am afraid the expense would be too great. My child seems to hear okay to me. Should I be concerned?*

A: Speech and hearing problems need to be identified very early. This is critical because hearing problems affect learning and language development in general. Your child could be at a serious disadvantage in school and at play. It is very important that potential problems such as this be recognized and resolved so that, in your particular case, your child has an equal chance to make the most of whatever life and school has to offer him. You should discuss the expense with your pediatrician and see if there is something that can be worked out; your child's hearing is too critical not to look for a solution. Your doctor will probably agree and try to help.

Q: *My baby is ten months old and doesn't have any teeth. Should I worry?*

A: Absolutely not. Although the average age for the first tooth is six months and the average child gets a tooth every month thereafter, many children are on different schedules. Just make sure that your child is developing in all other ways at a normal rate. Since the only problem you mentioned was teeth, I would look at this as an isolated factor and would not be concerned. Remember, not every child develops equally in every way. Some children speak sooner than others, some children grow faster than others, and some children's teeth come in quicker than others.

Q: *My doctor says that my child has thrush. What is that?*

A: *Thrush* is a yeast infection that affects the inside of the mouth. If you look inside your child's mouth, you see a whitish debris on the inside of the cheeks. This condition is relatively easy to treat. In most cases, it does not indicate a serious problem. If it ever recurs, however, you should see your pediatrician or family physician to have the problem treated.

Q: *My child is six months old, and we are going to the beach. How much time in the sun is appropriate for my baby?*

A: You should minimize the sun exposure as much as possible, especially at this age. Children get dehydrated quite easily. Make sure that your child is out of direct sunlight and that there is very little skin exposed to the sun. Talk to your doctor about a good sun screen. Some doctors approve of sun screens for infants, but others prefer that parents wait until their babies are older before they use them. Both arguments have merit, but the key is to limit your child's unnecessary exposure to the sun.

Q: *My child is in a day-care center and always seems to be getting sick. Do I have to take my child out of the center?*

A: Most people who use day-care centers for their children have no other option. In one respect, there are definite advantages to using day care. Many of the infections your child will undoubtedly get at some point in life occur earlier when the child is in day care, and he or she will therefore develop some resistance or immunity to them much sooner. If your child is constantly sick, however, you need to have him or her evaluated by your doctor to make sure that the child has no serious problems or diseases. Having runny noses, sore throats, ear infections, and coughs are part of growing up. Do not be overly concerned that you are endangering your children by placing them in a day-care center. Several studies have shown that children in day-care situations learn to interact quite well with other children at an early age and may even show advanced development over those who do not have such contact. There is no simple answer to your question, but if you are using a day-care center that is certified and that allows you access at any time of the day to see what is going on, you can be fairly confident that your child is not being exposed to serious diseases or physical danger. Apart from colds and the like, he or she is probably flourishing.

4

Colon Disorders and Cancer

Gerald J. Marks, M.D.

Historically, our understanding of the bowels and
their function has often been surrounded by mystery and mysticism.
Proper or improper elimination of the body's toxins, for which the bowels
are responsible, has been linked to many afflictions, from mental instability and spirit possession to poor eyesight or lusterless hair. In fact,
disorders of the gastrointestinal tract have contributed to the discomfort
and death of millions and have sometimes affected the course of history:
Painful hemorrhoids are said to have limited Napoleon's onslaught for
empire; the American stock market faltered with the diagnosis of President Ronald Reagan's colon cancer; and the world's Catholic population
prayed for the recovery of Pope John Paul II from colon surgery. Too
often, however, we ourselves or someone we know must contend with
an unpleasant affliction of the intestines. Through education and self-
awareness, we can achieve a better understanding of the way this system
of the body works and how to keep it working.

The Large Bowel (Colon and Rectum)

The architecture of the small and large intestines provides a remarkable
system for digesting food and separating waste from necessary nutrients.
The adult human small intestine can vary in length from twelve to twenty-two feet. This is where digested material is absorbed into the bloodstream. The large intestine, also known as the colon and rectum,

averages about five feet in length. It does the job of waste delivery or excretion. After nutrients are absorbed by the small intestine, the unabsorbed nutrients, fiber, water, and electrolytes, such as sodium, move into the colon. The main function of the colon is storage, which is aided by the absorption of water.

The large intestine makes strategic use of a limited space inside the body by winding up, over, and down, so waste can move relatively unimpeded. There are four parts to the large intestine. The first section, the *ascending colon*, starts on the right side of the abdomen in the cecum and moves up toward the liver. The second part, the *transverse colon*, provides a horizontal bridge from the ascending colon to the *descending colon*, the third section. The descending colon then moves into the *sigmoid*. Shaped like the letter **S**, the sigmoid colon curves toward the pelvis, where it joins the rectum, a relatively straight five-inch tube leading to the anus.

The sigmoid colon has a muscular action that is distinct, and the sigmoid is unlike the rest of the colon. This section is given to developing *diverticula*, which are pockets in the intestine that appear primarily in the sigmoid. Because it is far more active than the remainder of the colon, this area is also given to thickening, or *hypertrophy*, of the wall. Therefore, the sigmoid is often more susceptible to dysfunction.

The *sphincter* mechanism illustrates a biologic capability that is amazing in its function but not totally understood. This muscle at the lowest part of the rectum can discriminate between gas, fluid, and solid material. We generally do not appreciate its efficiency until it becomes impeded or fails to work.

The process of elimination in the colon illustrates an organized and efficient sanitation system—provided that adequate water is present, muscles are in good working order, the area is clear of infection, there are no congenital abnormalities, genetic factors are normal, and a person lives a relatively stress-free life. Unfortunately, one or more of these caveats are commonly called into question. As a result, certain disorders may result.

Disorders and Diagnoses

Any system that performs around-the-clock and as productively as the large bowel is always vulnerable to a variety of malfunctions. These glitches in production can be traced to anatomic disturbances, obstructions, external trauma, or diet.

Anatomic inadequacies refer to a change in the structure of this tube that carries out waste. Congenital abnormalities are infrequent. Generally, changes take place over time. Previous surgery may cause a lengthening in the structure that leaves space for *strictures,* or tight spots, to develop. As a result of inflammation from such diseases as ulcerative colitis, Crohn's disease, or diverticulitis, scarring produces a stricture that limits mobility in that area. A radiation injury inflicted during the treatment of a malignant condition somewhere in the abdomen can also leave behind scar tissue. The lowest form of a stricture is at the anal opening. Previous surgery that treated hemorrhoids or repaired an anal fissure can damage the sphincter's mechanism.

A *prolapsed rectum* occurs when the rectum falls out of position and protrudes painfully into the anus. Extraordinary straining or a traumatic situation engenders this embarrassing condition. The contents of the lower bowel cannot then be contained, causing the drainage of moisture. Although it is serious, a prolapsed rectum can be surgically treated. A prolapse may be hidden, or it may be obvious, where the rectum hangs out by itself. Many people with this condition must and do stay in bed.

A *mega colon* is another unusual transformation of the colon. Mega means big and, in this case, the colon becomes very wide in diameter as the result of long-standing constipation. When the bowel gets stretched, perhaps due to an impacted fecal mass, it loses its tone. Alternately, when the bowel elongates but then twists upon itself, it is called a *volvulus.* A person with a volvulus does not realize the anatomic change taking place but feels intense pain and cramping. This is an emergency situation that must be dealt with immediately. In certain cases, a volvulus may be manageable by the insertion of a tube, or it may require surgery.

People's diets frequently cause things to go wrong in their digestive systems. People do not always understand the relationship between certain foods and their bowels and that what they eat or drink can result in constipation or diarrhea. Some people cannot eat certain foods because of disturbances in their enzyme systems, the most common of which is a deficiency in lactase. *Lactase deficiency* produces an inability to process lactose—the essential enzyme in milk and all other dairy products. People with lactase deficiency may experience gas pains, stomach distention, and bloating and may have substantial diarrhea when they ingest lactose in milk, as well as in substances derived from milk, such as butter, cheese, ice cream, cakes made with those ingredients, and chocolate. Eating excess fruit, drinking excess fruit juice, or ingesting too much fiber or caffeine may also cause your body to produce *diarrhea*. Consuming unprocessed flour, such as that found in white bread, soft pretzels, or cakes, often leads to *constipation*.

Medications also affect the colon. Colchicine, a medication given for gout, may produce diarrhea in some people. Pain medications, such as morphine and morphine derivatives, may cause constipation. Certain antacids produce diarrhea, and others with calcium salts produce constipation. Drugs designed to control blood cholesterol also produce constipation. Some of these episodes can be quite severe. If you take too much antidiarrhea medication, you can experience great abdominal distention. It is important for all of us to understand what foods affect the functioning of our colons. You should adjust your diet if you find yourself suffering from diarrhea, constipation, or gas.

Obstructions in the bowel also interrupt the functioning of the intestines. They may be either *benign* (noncancerous) or *malignant* (cancerous). Unfortunately, the most common obstruction of the colon is a malignancy. Fortunately, a cancerous growth is almost always preceded by a benign polyp. If the polyp can be removed early and the area is monitored, cancer may be avoided. *Polyps* are abnormal growths rising from the lining of the large intestine (colon) and protruding into the intestinal canal. The growth of polyps is the most common condition affecting the colon and rectum, occurring in 15 percent to 20 percent of the adult population. They can be both diagnosed and removed through a *colonoscope,* a long flexible instrument that permits access to the entire colon.

It is important to remember that you should get a physical examination if you are experiencing any of the problems mentioned above. An examination involves palpation, or touching, of the abdomen, digital rectal examination, *anoscopy* (which uses a very small scope designed to look at the anus), *sigmoidoscopy* (which is an examination with a flexible fiberoptic sigmoidscope), a baseline barium enema with a colonoscopy, a CAT scan, and endorectal ultrasound or anal tenometry, which measures pressures and functions of the muscles. There are also means of studying the electrical activity of the muscles around the anal opening. A very special study, called the *dynamic defcogram,* videotapes the act of having a bowel movement. The patients ingests a mixture of barium and potato paste while sitting on a special X-ray machine that allows the function and ability of the sphincter muscle to be gauged. Physicians are now able to gain insight into certain problems that would otherwise go undiagnosed.

All of this may seem overwhelming at first. The emphasis, however, should be that there are many ways to diagnose and treat disorders of the colon and rectum. Testing is not a horrible experience. A gentle digital rectal exam is brief and painless. The scope used for the sigmoidoscopy is a thin, flexible, fiberoptic tube that shows the physician the lower one-fourth to one-third of the colon. The exam may be a bit unnerving for some people, but it is certainly not painful when it is done properly. The examination can be conducted with minimal preparation in a physician's office, frequently in less than two minutes.

Colonoscopy uses a longer flexible instrument and usually permits inspection of the entire colon. Bowel preparation is required and sedation is often used. The colon can also be indirectly examined using barium enema X-ray techniques. This examination uses a barium solution to coat the colon lining and accommodate X-ray images.

As a caution, perhaps too many people rely on the *hemoccult slide test* as a diagnostic screening test. This is the home kit that you can use to collect onto a special slide a stool sample and mail it off to a laboratory for testing. This test is used to assist evaluation of rectal bleeding. People often rely solely upon the hemoccult test as an indicator for malignant conditions; yet it has a high false-negative rate. A recent study reported in the *Journal of the American Medical Association* indicates that most cancers and the vast majority of polyps will be missed if this test alone is used.

Symptoms

Some symptoms may have substantial meaning, and some may be of absolutely no consequence. For example, some degree of bloating follows certain dietary indiscretions. Even diarrhea or constipation may be a temporary response to an unfamiliar factor, such as diet, increased stress, bacteria, or a virus. It is important to keep in mind, however, that these symptoms may also herald the beginning of a more invasive condition that requires attention. Again, you are your own best judge. Everyone feels irregular from time to time, but if that irregularity becomes, in a sense, regular, you must adjust the circumstances to be rid of it. That means altering diet, taking note of changes, and going to the doctor.

The large bowel has no sensation; it can only perceive an increase in pressure. As the muscle of the bowels work against this increase in pressure, the brain registers the activity as cramps. *Cramps* can be felt as a nonlocalized, encompassing sensation in the abdomen. Cramping pain is generally colicky, meaning that it is not constant but comes in waves. When sharp pangs are felt, the colon is generally not responsible. True pain arises from the *peritoneal envelope,* the membrane that lines the abdominal cavity and covers the stomach, intestines, and abdominal organs. If that pain is constant, it is probably an inflammation of the peritoneum, indicating appendicitis or peritonitis.

Blood may be present in the stool because of a few different conditions, the least serious of which is hemorrhoids and the most serious of which is a possible cancer in the colon or rectum. Rectal bleeding may be the result of inflammation from certain diseases, such as Crohn's disease or ulcerative colitis, or it may originate higher up in the colon, which indicates a greater problem. In any case, bleeding requires careful evaluation. At the very least the patient must know that the physician consulted must do a digital rectal examination, plus or minus an anoscopy, and, certainly, a sigmoidoscopic examination. For individuals older than age thirty-five, examination should be supplemented by a barium enema study. If these measures fail to explain the cause of the bleeding, especially if the patient has a family history of colorectal problems or colon cancer, he or she should have further testing and a colonoscopy.

When the abdomen feels unnaturally full, it may not be from a recent meal. Bloating or distention fills the intestines the way air fills a tire. This condition may be exhibited by cramping or even flatulence. Generally, a person who becomes briefly, albeit uncomfortably, bloated has eaten a food that is not agreeable to the digestive tract, so the gas problem's cause may be inconsequential. Alternately, however, bloating may indicate a more serious problem, and if it persists, you should definitely consult your physician.

Fever originating in the colon is sometimes associated with abdominal pain. Both are indicators that the large intestine is undergoing bombardment by irregular invaders. Infectious diarrhea and diseases of inflammation, such as ulcerative colitis and diverticulitis, can aggravate the structure of the colon. Just as the body can sense any foreign body or substance within it, so, too, does the colon respond by becoming inflamed, thus hot and feverish, when it is irritated.

The preponderance of air in the colon and rectum, which is often released as flatulence, is a result of the air we swallow. It also may be the result of eating certain food, such as excessive carbohydrates like beans.

People who have a *lactose intolerance* probably notice increased gas after they ingest milk products. Additionally, it is likely that, as people age, their ability to handle various foodstuffs changes and the production of gas becomes commonplace.

Diarrhea and constipation may be a purely functional matter or may herald the presence of a benign or malignant tumor. Obstructions that may irritate the sidewall of the bowel sometimes produce diarrhea. If the diarrhea persists, this must be brought to the attention of your physician. Again, the patient should be aware of what a proper examination entails. Simply by performing a digital rectal examination and an examination of the abdomen the doctor may be able to determine clues to the disorder.

Functional Disturbances

Some types of malfunction in the colon are commonplace and should not be viewed as a function-altering prospects. Basically, the bowel may be reacting to conditions that can be explained by particulars of diet or merely by the lack of sufficient fluid.

For instance, diarrhea and constipation are familiar to most people. Although they are usually temporary and benign situations, diarrhea or constipation may be indicators of a more serious ailment. The best way to gauge whether a problem exists is to recognize your own pattern of bowel movements—anywhere from one movement to three movements a day, or just four a week, may be normal. The term *constipation* is derived from the Latin word *constipatus,* which means "to press or crowd together; to pack; to cram." Consequently, constipation occurs when a clogged bowel makes evacuation difficult. In contrast, *diarrhea* is characterized by overly frequent evacuation, with loose, watery stools. Both conditions may result from stress or from poor diet. Low intake of roughage causes constipation, and eating excess amounts of prunes or beans contributes to diarrhea, as does overuse of laxatives or taking certain medications. Emotional stress and tension may also produce diarrhea or constipation. When stress generates rapid digestive activity, it can cause the well-known nervous "butterflies," and it can affect the bowel, causing diarrhea. If stress manifests as a spasm in the bowel, constipation is the result. If constipation persists for two weeks with no relief or if diarrhea lasts for more than forty-eight hours, you should consult your doctor. Any noticeable change in bowel habits should be evaluated by your physician.

Conditions such as lactose intolerance can be especially insidious because there is lactose in so many substances, such as chocolate, rich cookies, cakes, and cheese. In addition, some people's digestive systems cannot handle certain foods like wheat, egg whites, or corn. Food idiosyncrasies can often be found to explain a lot of people's bowel problems, but they must first be recognized.

Sometimes, disorders in the digestive tract cannot be traced to any particular condition, but knowledge of that fact does little to reduce the very real discomfort a person may be experiencing. In such cases, *irritable bowel syndrome* (IBS) is credited as the culprit. IBS is a condition that is ill-defined, and the diagnosis is overused. People who experience cramping pain as a result of hyperactivity of the colon are commonly told they have IBS. Many of these people, I believe, have unrecognized lactose intolerance. Many of them may also have functional disturbances as a result of irregular activity in the sigmoid colon, which is associated with diverticular disease.

Again, diet should be suspected: Caffeine stimulates the colon, as can too much fruit. Beer, whiskey, wine, and other alcoholic beverages are acknowledged as aggravating the function of the bowels in some people. Always keep in mind the possible effect of certain medications. Eating a low-fat, high-fiber diet is acknowledged as the most effective deterrent to bowel troubles.

Disease States

Although the workings of the bowels are a fascinating cooperation of structure, process, and components, their complicated engineering can malfunction as a result of only slight adjustments. I have discussed anatomic and dietary factors, but disease is perhaps the most prevalent problem that affects the intestines.

Benign but Inflammatory

The colon harbors an abundance of bacteria, but these organisms serve a purpose; the colon will tolerate few invaders. When bacteria or viruses infiltrate the colon or rectum, they react by becoming inflamed. *Infectious diarrhea,* a viral diarrhea, is one culprit. Although it is familiar to adult and youth intestinal tracts, the virus can cause colon inflammation and it can agitate the respiratory system. Bacteria that cause diarrhea often affect travelers, who may pick them up from eating improperly cooked or stored food or from drinking infected water. It is possible to become infected by bacteria locally, through poor sanitation. *E. coli,* a major bacterial agent, is nothing more than an overgrowth of a normal organism that leads to intestinal distress.

A person may have *diverticulosis,* which occurs when small, saclike swellings called *diverticula* form along the wall of the colon. There seems to be some connection between diverticular disease and the Western diet, which is low in fiber content. (Diverticulitis rarely occurs in Africa and Asia, where more fiber is consumed.) Diverticula are present in 30 percent to 40 percent of persons over age fifty, with increasing incidence for each subsequent decade of life. The resulting symptoms may be minor: cramping pains with tenderness in the left side of the abdomen; small, hard bowel movements with occasional attacks of diarrhea. When the diverticula bleed, bright red blood passes in the stools. Only when these sacs become inflamed and cause the disease *diverticulitis* do definite symptoms of severe abdominal pain, nausea, and fever develop. Your physician will probably order blood and stool samples, an endoscopic exam, and a barium enema to rule out cancer of the large intestine, which has similar symptoms. Diverticulitis is treatable; it may even be prevented if you maintain a diet of whole grain breads, oatmeal or bran cereals, and plenty of fibrous fresh fruits and vegetables.

Ulcerative colitis generally involves just the rectum or sigmoid. This condition causes a reaction opposite to that of diverticulitis on the colon. Instead of sacs protruding from the colon wall, small ulcers or abscesses form on the inner lining of the colon. This condition is relatively rare and is diagnosed by measures similar to those for diverticulitis. *Ulcerative colitis* is more common in women and is likely to develop between ages fifteen and thirty-five. It is a chronic condition that tends to lead to an increased risk of colon cancer after ten years. Symptoms may be very mild and unnoticeable and may recur over a period of years. In severe cases, there may be pain in the lower abdomen, which is relieved with a bowel movement; fever, weight loss, joint pain, and an attack of painful diarrhea with blood, pus, and mucus in it. If it just involves the rectum, *proctitis* is the name given to the condition. *Radiation colitis* can be generated by external radiation that is given at high doses to control cancer at various sites in the abdomen.

Crohn's disease has an unknown origin, but it does seem to run in some families. It has been a rare disorder in the Western world, but it is gradually becoming more common. There are about twice as many cases of it today as there were twenty years ago. Crohn's disease causes periodic attacks of cramps, lower right abdominal pain, diarrhea, a slight fever, and nausea. The small intestine is most commonly involved, although swelling can reach into the colon. Medication and nutrition can help control the symptoms. Since the ability to absorb adequate nutrients often is limited in people with Crohn's disease, your physician may advise vitamin B_{12} and a low-fat diet to assist absorption. Surgery is prescribed in 70 percent of cases.

If the inflamed intestinal wall leaks because of untreated Crohn's disease, the more serious condition peritonitis may occur. Almost always due to an underlying disease, *peritonitis* is inflammation of the membrane that lines the abdominal cavity and covers the stomach, intestines, and abdominal organs. Pain is severe and unexpected, sometimes causing nausea and vomiting. As the pain decreases, the area may swell. The condition will not subside on its own, however, and should be treated immediately. Peritonitis is not likely to occur if medical help is sought before symptoms progress to an emergency situation. For instance, peritonitis may arise from untreated appendicitis. Many people do not associate the *appendix* with the digestive tract, but it is a thin, little pouch that extends off the first part of the colon. In humans, the appendix has no real function, and it can become diseased. If you have severe pain on the right side of the abdomen, you may be having an attack of *appendicitis*, which afflicts one in five hundred people every year. The infection may result in surgery to remove the diseased appendix.

Neoplasms and Tumors

Cancer of the colon and rectum is the most common internal malignancy that affects men and women in eastern Pennsylvania and New Jersey; it is the second most common cancer in the remainder of the country. *Colorectal cancer* is the only visceral cancer that is preceded by a benign but premalignant condition such as a polyp. Polyps can be readily identified and removed by colonoscopic intervention, thereby interrupting the growth of a cancer. This situation allows the potential for great rates of prevention of tumors of the colon and rectum, but only through heightened participation by individuals.

Individuals interested in their colon health should have a flexible sigmoidoscopic examination by age forty, or forty-five if you do not have additional risk factors. It would also be appropriate to have a barium enema. The sigmoidoscopic examination should be repeated in five years, followed by two- or three-year intervals. After age fifty, annual exams are desired because risk increases with age. Seventy percent of the part of the colon and rectum that gives rise to cancer is examined during the brief interval of a sigmoidoscopic examination.

For the longest time, colorectal cancer has been the unmentionable cancer. People would not talk about it because they felt uncomfortable discussing this area of the body and uncertain about what could be done for them. Today, we know that 98 percent to 100 percent of these cancers can be cured when they are detected early. Even for the more advanced tumors, an aggressive program of combination therapy has been able to achieve an 80 percent, five-year, cure rate. Preservation of sphincter function—the ability of a person to pass stools without the use of a colostomy bag—has been a priority in treatment.

Fear of *colostomy* (an opening to the outside world through the abdominal wall) has kept people from seeking attention for their symptoms. These days, rarely is a "bag" required for someone who has had a colon tumor removed. Even rectal tumors, which are closer to the anus and pose a more severe threat to function, can be removed without permanent damage. That is the good news; the bad news is that the incidence of these tumors continues to rise.

In Western countries, the colon and rectum account for more new cases of cancer each year than does any other anatomic site except the lung. The American Cancer Society estimated that 109,000 new cases of colon cancer would be diagnosed in 1993, with 57,000 deaths. Rectal cancer was projected to afflict 43,000 Americans, with 7,000 deaths. Colon cancer accounts for about 20 percent of the deaths due to malignant disease in this country.

The key to improving statistics on this disease is to get people into the doctor as soon as they start experiencing symptoms, if not before. Ideally, screening methods will detect those people at risk of colorectal cancer so that they can be monitored. If you have a family member who has had cancer of either the colon or the rectum, you are immediately at an increased risk. Colorectal cancers may begin to grow without symptoms. You must be conscious, however, of such symptoms as rectal bleeding, altered bowel habits, abdominal cramps or pain, blood in the stool, unexplained anemia, and unexplained weight loss.

An individual with these symptoms deserves to be investigated completely. That means a physical examination of the abdomen, digital rectal examination, sigmoidoscopic examination, and then a baseline barium enema or a colonoscopy, depending upon other risk factors. The patient has the right to request these tests; a superficial examination is not enough.

Anorectal Problems

People commonly experience *hemorrhoids*. These prominent veins in the anus are generally not painful unless the blood in the dilated vein becomes clotted. The American diet of highly refined food products is partly to blame for this disorder. The location of the hemorrhoid causes difficulty because the pressure of sitting and persistent straining to have a bowel movement may cause the hemorrhoid to rupture, and thus bleeding occurs.

Hemorrhoids are annoying and uncomfortable but they also are common and treatable. Again, a change in diet usually makes a difference: Eat plenty of fresh fruit, vegetables, and whole grain or bran cereals and bread, and drink sufficient quantities of water. A sitz bath—sitting in plain warm water for about ten minutes—can also provide some relief. In cases of severe, persistent pain, your physician may elect to remove the hemorrhoid containing the clot with a small incision. The procedure is performed under local anesthesia as an outpatient, and it generally provides immediate relief.

Other dysfunctions in the anus that may cause bleeding are anal fissures and fistulas. A *fissure* is a break in the lining of the anal canal that occurs just at the outer edge of the opening. It is the result of tightness in the wall and overstretching by a hard, large stool. It is more common in women and often heals after one adds fiber to the diet. *Fistulas* are abnormal tubelike passageways from the canal to a hole in the skin. These result from abscesses beneath the lining of the rectum and generally require surgery. Both fissures and fistulas require medical attention, for treatment as well as to rule out other conditions. Fistulas sometimes indicate the presence of Crohn's disease, the chronic inflammatory condition of the digestive tract discussed above.

Improved Treatment

Physicians and researchers have made some important observations over the past fifteen or so years in the management of colorectal cancers. We have been able nearly to double the survival rate. High-dose, preoperative radiation therapy for select cancers can reduce the incidence of local failure, virtually double the survival rate, and make the need for a permanent colostomy rare. In the past, a tumor was surgically removed, along with an extensive portion of the colon so that function would be inhibited. Today, there are many options for adjunctive therapy: Radiation can be administered prior to, during, or following surgery to reduce the number of cancer cells; chemotherapy helps to clear the area of residual cancer; and new knowledge about genetic therapy is prompting some to propose it as another potential treatment.

The colonoscopy is typically used to remove polyps in the colon. This outpatient procedure allows for rapid recovery and reduces the possibility of future tumors. Once polyps become malignant or cancer develops somewhere along the colon or rectum, surgery becomes necessary. Surgical access to the pelvis was historically limited because of its funnel shape. About eighteen years ago, surgical experience, coupled with strides being made in radiation oncology and special surgical techniques, helped physicians to determine that high-dose, preoperative radiation could shrink the tumor to a manageable point. Next, the special surgical techniques could be used to approach the colon and rectum in a manner that more easily exposed the affected area. Now, cancerous tumors even in the lowest part of the rectum may be removed completely with little incidence of recurrence and with sphincter function maintained.

An integral part of the success in treating colorectal tumors is due to the cooperation maintained among the various specialists. Obviously, your surgeon should be working closely with a radiation oncologist, but I also like to emphasize the importance of sharing expertise with medical oncologists, radiologists, even urologists or gynecologists. There is no reason to exclude input from the various experts involved in your care.

Although statistics indicate that the location of colorectal tumors seems to be shifting to lower in the rectum, that should not raise the specter of colostomy in a patient's mind. It is true that there has been an inordinately high rate of local recurrences of rectal cancers, often ruling out restorative surgery in the rectum. But sphincter preservation can be accomplished in cancers even near the anus if high-dose preoperative radiation is administered.

Contrary to former therapies, physicians are also realizing that they do not have to rush into surgery when a tumor is discovered. Even waiting a month and a half after radiation therapy does not affect the outcome. In fact, it allows the irradiated tissue to strengthen so that it is not damaged during surgery. An artificial opening after the surgery is often required, but only on a temporary basis.

In treatment for cancers of the colon and rectum, quality of life need not be compromised. Physicians know from the growing success of therapy that we have refined care almost to a routine procedure. This experience can help us to begin to prevent more malignancies. Screening is a primary factor in cancer prevention. Diet is another consideration. All facts point to high-fiber, low-fat foods as a buffer against intestinal disease. Some studies suggest that regular doses of aspirin reduce the likelihood of bowel cancers. Your family history can also give you information about your risk potential. Basically, having self-awareness and awareness about the diseases that affect your digestive system is the best way to take charge of your colon health.

Genetic Defects

A primary goal in informing people about gastrointestinal disease, especially colorectal cancer, is to encourage them to recognize when they are at risk so that they can take steps to protect themselves. Long ago, the medical community determined that there is a genetic link to cancers of the colon. Thanks to ongoing colorectal genetic studies, the medical establishment now knows that certain gene defects are responsible for inherited forms of colon cancer. This finding may lead to quicker diagnoses and could save thousands of lives. For example, researchers at Johns Hopkins University found that a mutated gene, carried by about one in every two hundred people in the Western world, identifies people with an inherited and extraordinarily high risk of the disease. The gene defect is thought to be responsible for about one in every seven colon cancer cases. Hopkins's scientists also found that a gene defect that is responsible for inherited colon cancer also plays a major role in the development of the more common, nonhereditary colon cancers.

Genetic studies are aimed at allowing doctors the ability to target colorectal tumors by finding genetic markers, thus locating tumors before they can be visually detected. This type of cooperation between scientists and clinicians is a major emphasis in the future treatment of cancers in the colon and rectum. In addition, the near future holds the development of synthetic peptides that can be injected directly into the tumor to block the proliferation of malignant cells. Already, researchers are designing computer-assisted programs to develop new cancer drugs, and doctors are taking the inspection of tumors more and more from the bedside into the laboratory in order to better gauge the molecular basis of tumor existence and to help save lives.

About the Author

Dr. Gerald J. Marks, director of the division of colorectal surgery at Thomas Jefferson University Hospital, Philadelphia, is an internationally renowned colorectal surgeon. In his capacities as professor of surgery for Jefferson Medical College and director of the Comprehensive Rectal Cancer Center, Dr. Marks has developed a standard of care in the treatment of colorectal disease that is maintained both academically and clinically.

A pioneer in colonoscopy and polypectomy, Dr. Marks used the first production-model colonoscope in the country in 1969. He later pioneered the use of the flexible fiberoptic sigmoidoscope.

Dr. Marks is a graduate of Jefferson Medical College and has been involved in the surgical care of diseases of the colon and rectum for more than four decades. He has published extensively in medical books and professional journals on colorectal surgical research. In addition, Dr. Marks has served as an officer in various medical societies and has provided editorial input into such publications as the New England Journal of Medicine *and* Diseases of the Colon and Rectum. *He is senior editor of* Surgical Endoscopy, Ultrasound, and Interventional Techniques. *He has functioned as a liaison for the world medical teaching community, by sharing his expertise with various European centers in Italy and Germany, and in Israel, other Middle Eastern countries, and countries of the Far East.*

QUESTIONS FOR THE DOCTOR

Q: Do hemorrhoids lead to cancer?
A: No. There is no relationship between hemorrhoids and cancer. The symptoms of hemorrhoids, particularly bleeding, are similar to those of colorectal cancer and other diseases of the digestive system, however. It is important to have all of your symptoms investigated by a physician specially trained in treating diseases of the colon and rectum. Do not rely on over-the-counter medications or other self-treatments.

Q: *Do polyps need to be treated?*
A: Since there is no foolproof way to predict whether a polyp is or will become malignant, total removal of all polyps is advised. The vast majority of polyps can be removed by snaring them with a wire loop passed through a colonoscope. Small polyps can be destroyed simply by touching them with a coagulating electrical current.

Q: *If my father or mother had colorectal cancer, at what point in my life should I be evaluated?*
A: The American Cancer Society recommends that a digital rectal examination be performed annually from age forty, with a sigmoidoscopic examination, every three to five years after age fifty. However, beginning at age forty-five with endoscopic examination can be more beneficial. These measures are for everyone, even those without increased risk of developing cancer. But if someone in your family has been diagnosed with colorectal cancer, you are definitely at an increased risk and should begin screening at age thirty-five.

Q: *I have pain in my chest every time I take a drink of alcohol. Is this all in my head (my parents are adamant against drinking alcohol) or do I have a problem?*
A: Certainly you can "wish" yourself to have a problem, but in most cases the chest pain you are describing is heartburn. There is a long tube called the esophagus that connects your mouth to your stomach, and it does not tolerate stomach acid very well, so when acid from your stomach travels up into the esophagus you may experience symptoms similar to chest pain. All of us have a valve at the top of the stomach to block the release of acid, but many times it doesn't work. Certain foods, such as chili peppers, can cause an increase of acid and so can caffeine, smoking, aspirin products, and alcohol. Often, all it takes is an antacid to relieve the problem, but if it continues over a period of time, you may need prescription medications. One thing that may help is to raise the head of your bed, because gravity might keep the acid in the stomach. In your case, it might be the alcohol that is setting off your problem. Remember, there are many causes of chest pain, and, certainly, we have to consider heart disease whenever chest pain is encountered. Although the chest pain is usually quite different from heartburn, make sure you see a physician if you have any questions at all.

Q: *I have pain in my stomach on the right side and I seem to get it every time I eat fried food. I also burp a lot and I am embarrassed by it. Do you know what this could be?*

A: Obviously, we can't make a diagnosis without seeing you, but you might want to have your physician examine your gallbladder. The gallbladder can become a source of problems for people when the ducts that supply it become obstructed. This can be made worse by eating fried, fatty foods. Gallbladder trouble seems to occur in overweight men and women more than in thin men and women, and pregnant women often experience its symptoms. A buildup of gas can lead to belching. Surgery can now be performed through the laparoscope. In many cases, gallbladder surgery is far easier to go through than it used to be. You should check with your doctor about the pain and gas you are having. If the problem is your gallbladder and it becomes infected, it can lead to serious problems.

5

Diabetes

José F. Caro, M.D., and
Rishi Rastogi, M.D.

To understand diabetes, you need to understand how food is digested. After you eat, your stomach digests the food, or breaks it down into glucose, amino acids (from protein), or triglycerides. These substances are then absorbed through the intestine to reach the blood. The amino acids can also be converted into glucose, if it is needed by the body. The glucose in the blood causes the pancreas (a small organ that sits behind the stomach) to secrete insulin. Insulin helps glucose get into the body's cells (through specific areas present on the cell surface, called "insulin receptors"); once inside the cells, the glucose serves as body fuel to provide energy.

As you eat, the glucose level in the blood goes up, and this glucose causes the B-cells of the pancreas to secrete insulin. If insulin is working properly, the glucose enters the cells and the glucose level in the blood goes down. If the pancreas is making the right amount of insulin, the glucose level is normally maintained within a narrow range of 80 milligrams to 140 milligrams per deciliter. So, food makes the glucose level go up and insulin makes the glucose level come down as glucose leaves the blood and enters the cells.

Diabetes mellitus is a disorder of the body's metabolism that causes high blood sugar. It is caused by either an absolute deficiency of insulin secretion from the B-cells of the pancreas (Type I diabetes mellitus) or by resistance to the insulin's action because the insulin receptors are not working properly (Type II diabetes mellitus). (See Table 5–1 for the ma-

TABLE 5-1
Comparison of Type I and Type II Diabetes Mellitus

	Type I	Type II
Prevalence	10–20%	80–90%
Age	younger individuals or nonobese adults	obese adults
Insulin reserve	decreased or absent	normal or high
Islet cell antibodies	usually present	absent
Probable cause	infection or toxic insult to pancreatic B-cells in genetically predisposed persons	decreased sensitivity of insulin receptors to insulin action
Onset	childhood or early adulthood	around age forty
Treatment	diet and insulin (insulin required for survival)	diet, exercise, and weight reduction, and sometimes oral medications; may occasionally need insulin
Concordance in identical twins	<50%	close to 100%
Ketoacidosis*	can be marked	absent
Race	usually Caucasians or population with white genetic admixture	all populations
Familial aggregation	uncommon	very common

*Ketoacidosis: using body fat instead of glucose as fuel, leading to increased activity in the blood and dehydration.

jor distinctions between Type I and Type II diabetes mellitus.) Diabetes mellitus is diagnosed by identifying elevated blood glucose concentrations after an overnight fast, by finding concentrations greater than 140 mg/dl on at least two occasions, or by performing an oral glucose tolerance test.

The elevated blood glucose may be found during a routine blood test. Sometimes the symptoms of high blood glucose are present at the time of diagnosis. The symptoms of diabetes include increased thirst, weight loss, increased appetite, blurring of vision, increased urination, and tingling and numbness of hands and feet.

In *Type I diabetes,* the B-cells (the cells that make insulin) start to die off; the reason for this is not clear. Some people probably have a predisposition to develop diabetes, and when they contract some viral infection or suffer some kind of toxic insult, their bodies produce antibodies (substances that normally fight any infection), which attack the body's own B-cells and destroy them. The B-cells start to die long before any symptoms appear, however. Since the pancreas of people with Type I diabetes makes very little or no insulin, this substance must be supplied, in the form of injections, to control blood glucose levels. People with Type I diabetes must learn how to balance their meals (both amount and timing), their physical activities, and their insulin injections. One needs to match the peak level of insulin with the peak level of blood glucose.

Type II diabetes is the most common type of diabetes. It tends to run in families, but the exact mode of inheritance is not known. If many people in your family have diabetes, it is more likely that you will also develop diabetes, especially if it is present in both maternal and paternal sides of the family. In Type II diabetes the body is still able to make insulin, but the insulin cannot work properly because of the problem in the cells' insulin receptors.

Type II diabetes usually appears around age forty. Symptoms may start gradually, so it is harder to identify than Type I. Many people with Type II diabetes are overweight and may also have high blood pressure and high serum cholesterol. The presence of diabetes accelerates the progression of *atherosclerosis* (hardening and narrowing of the arteries), which can give rise to an increase in the incidence of heart attack, stroke, and gangrene in the feet. The coexistence of high blood pressure and cigarette smoking may further aggravate the problem.

Type II diabetes can be treated with diet control and weight reduction. The weight reduction is the most important part of the management, because it will not only help to control the diabetes but will also help to prevent high blood pressure, high serum cholesterol, and atherosclerosis. Sometimes, early atherosclerosis can be reversed by weight reduction, and this will help to decrease the chances of developing a heart attack, a stroke, or another vascular complication. If, after adequate diet control and weight reduction, blood glucose is still high, then oral medications are given. Most Type II diabetics do not need insulin; only very few people require it.

The goal in the treatment of diabetes is to try to keep the blood glucose levels within a normal range and to prevent wide fluctuations. A low level of blood glucose (hypoglycemia) can cause symptoms such as confusion, impaired thinking, nausea, sweating, hunger, and heart palpitations. Severe hypoglycemia may cause epileptic seizures and coma. A high level of blood glucose (hyperglycemia) can cause dehydration with ketoacidosis (using body fat instead of glucose as fuel) in Type I diabetics, if they have not taken insulin, and severe dehydration with coma in Type

II diabetics. Death can occur in either situation if the patient is not treated promptly.

Complications in Diabetes

Both types of diabetics can develop certain complications involving the eyes, kidneys, nerves, blood vessels, skin, and other organs. This chapter looks at each of these in detail.

Eye Disease

In the eyes, the small blood vessel involvement caused by diabetes can cause microaneurysms (out-pouching of the wall of smaller blood vessels), hemorrhages, and swelling of the retina (inner coat of eyeball), causing impaired vision. This is called *background retinopathy*. In *proliferative retinopathy*, which is more common in Type I diabetics, there is blockage of the small vessels and abnormal growth of the neighboring blood vessels. Later, this can cause hemorrhaging and detachment of the retina, resulting in blindness. Patients with this condition are treated with laser surgery. Both types of diabetics can also develop cataracts, which develop more rapidly in people with uncontrolled diabetes who have high blood glucose. For patients who have had diabetes for more than five years, a yearly eye examination is recommended to detect early eye disease.

Kidney Disease

The small blood vessel involvement can also cause kidney disease, where there is spillage of protein in the urine. This is called *diabetic nephropathy*, and in advanced stages patients may develop high blood pressure, swelling of the body, and high serum cholesterol levels. These patients may ultimately become dependent on dialysis. Early stages of kidney involvement can be detected by spillage of smaller amounts of protein (called microalbuminuria). If this is found, it can be treated by good blood glucose control, a low protein diet, and medication. These steps may be able to reverse early kidney disease.

Nervous System Disease

The nervous system involvement in diabetes is called *diabetic neuropathy*. It can show up as tingling and numbness of hands and feet, foot drop or wrist drop, problems with blood pressure control, rapid pulse, diarrhea, and impotence. These problems can be managed by various means but they are often irreversible. Patients with impotence can now use penile implants. Patients with sensory loss in the feet should be particularly careful about their feet, and should see a podiatrist from time to time. They should wear properly fitted shoes and stockings and should avoid foot friction or pressure. They should file their nails carefully with an emery board, and they should never cut the corners of their nails.

Heart Disease

The small blood vessel involvement in the heart can cause a dilation or enlargement of the heart called *cardiomyopathy.* The large blood vessel involvement can cause accelerated atherosclerosis. Disease of the large blood vessels supplying the heart can cause heart attack, which is three to five times more common in diabetics than in nondiabetics. An important feature of this type of heart attack is that pain may not be felt at all, because the nerves carrying the pain sensations are damaged.

Large blood vessel involvement of the legs can cause gangrene (infection, rot) of the feet. These patients may also have *diabetic peripheral neuropathy* present, in the form of numbness of the feet. Prevention of any foot injury is very important. These patients should not smoke and should avoid certain medications, which may further reduce the blood flow to the feet. A diabetic who develops foot ulcers should seek medical attention immediately. Blood flow in the legs can be measured by certain tests (Doppler, ultrasound) and blood flow can be improved by surgery (endarterectomy and bypass operations).

Infections

Certain types of infections, for example, urinary tract infections, yeast infections of the vagina and esophagus, infection of the foot bones (osteomyelitis), and ear infections, are more common in diabetics than in nondiabetics. All diabetics must pay closer attention to their health.

Managing Diabetes

There are several ways to attack diabetes. *Diet therapy* is the most important part of the management of both types of diabetes. If you are a diabetic, the number of calories (i.e., the amount of food) you require depends on your body size, whether or not you need to reduce weight (as most Type II diabetics should), your lifestyle, and your daily activities.

The timing of your meals and snacks is very important. Particularly if you are taking insulin, you should try to match each mealtime rise in blood glucose with the insulin "peak effect." The kind of food you eat is also important. Certain foods, for example, candy, chocolate, honey, ice cream, cakes, and most desserts may cause rapid increases in blood glucose, too rapid for the insulin to work effectively. These foods should be curtailed. Your best choices are fruits, vegetables, cereals and whole-grain breads, low-fat dairy products (skim milk, cottage cheese, and low-fat yogurt), and low-fat meats. The fat intake should be 35 percent or less of total calories. Complex carbohydrates may be consumed liberally and should contribute as much as 50 percent of the total calories. The saturated fat should be reduced to one-third of total daily intake, and cholesterol should be restricted to less than 300 mg per day.

Dietary fiber should be added to the diets of all diabetics. The fiber that is found in bran, beans, oatmeal, or apple skin is indigestible. When diabetics eat this kind of fiber, the intestinal transit time is increased, causing slower absorption of glucose and thereby decreasing hyperglycemia. Only noncaloric sweeteners, such as saccharin, should be used by diabetics, despite the potential risk of bladder cancer from their long-term use. Other relatively safe sweeteners are aspartame, sorbitol (which may cause diarrhea), and fructose. The American Diabetes Association offers free pamphlets with dietary information.

Exercise is very important in the management of diabetes. Exercise is an excellent means of weight reduction, which is crucial for the obese Type II diabetic. Exercise and weight reduction increase the effectiveness of insulin and are an excellent means of improving utilization of fat and carbohydrates. Strenuous exercise can, however, precipitate hypoglycemia (low blood sugar), and patients should know how to prevent this type of situation. Diabetics often inject insulin into the stomach, because the site of insulin injection should be far away from the muscles most involved in exercise, otherwise, rapid absorption of insulin may also precipitate hypoglycemia. A decrease in a diabetic's weight will also decrease his or her need for insulin or oral medications. If you do lose weight, you should check with your doctor to prevent the overtreatment of insulin and hypoglycemia.

Exercise is helpful not only for the diabetes but also for improving or reducing your chances of having a stroke, heart attack, peripheral vascular disease, and kidney disease. The degree of weight reduction you need depends upon your present weight. A combination of caloric restriction, exercise, and consistent good eating habits is required for a successful weight-reduction program, but a lot depends on the motivation of the patient and the enthusiasm of the health care team. Many people are able to reduce their weight but find it hard to keep their weight down for a long time, so consistent reinforcement from the health care team is necessary.

Medication can benefit those with diabetes who do not need to take insulin. Oral medications of the group "sulfonylurea" are useful for Type II diabetics. Some common ones are Tolbutamide (Orinase), Tolazamide (Tolinase), Chlorpropamide (Diabinese), Gliburide (DiaBeta, Micronase), and Glipizide (Glucotrol). These medications act by increasing the release of insulin from the B-cells of the pancreas and by increasing insulin binding to the insulin receptors. These medications are not useful for Type I diabetic patients, because these drugs require functioning pancreatic B-cells to produce their effect on blood glucose. They are most appropriate for use by the nonobese Type II patient whose hyperglycemia has not responded to diet therapy alone. They are also useful for obese Type II diabetics (who usually have peripheral insensitivity to circulating insulin) when weight reduction and diet therapy have been inadequate for blood glucose control. For hyperglycemia in obese Type II diabetics, which can be very severe, these agents may be used in the beginning of the management to improve blood glucose control, until other concurrent measures (for example, diet, exercise, and weight reduction) can sustain the improvement without the need for oral drugs.

Insulin therapy is mandatory for all Type I diabetics and is also indicated for those Type II diabetics whose hyperglycemia does not respond to diet therapy, weight reduction, and oral medication. The older insulins obtained from pork or beef have higher incidences of allergic reaction and resistance. Newer, highly purified, human insulin, however, is now manufactured commercially by a biosynthetic technique, employing recombinant DNA, and has a much lower incidence of insulin allergy, immune insulin resistance, and local reactions at injection sites. The different types of insulin are classified as short-acting (regular insulin), intermediate-acting (NPH and Lente insulin), and long-acting insulin (ultralente and protamine zinc insulin). They have different onsets of action, peak effect, and duration of action. (A premixed combination of regular and NPH, called Novolin 70/30 or Humulin 70/30, is also available.)

The conventional insulin therapy consists of combinations of short-acting or intermediate-acting and long-acting insulin. The insulin injections are given simultaneously, away from the exercising muscle. The timing of the insulin injections and the timing of meals are planned in such a way that the peak effect of insulin action matches the maximum increase in blood glucose level. Insulin is given as a single shot or as multiple shots during the day, depending on the patient. The most widely used concentration of insulin is 100U/ml, but other concentrations are also available.

Ideally, insulin treatment of Type I diabetes is started in the hospital, particularly for children, because the patient's initial requirement of insulin can vary a great deal. The hospital also provides a protected environment in which the patient's insulin levels can be closely monitored and blood glucose insulin requirements can be determined efficiently. During the hospital stay, the patient can build up confidence and learn about the new disease, blood glucose testing, diet, and hypoglycemia. Later, blood glucose monitoring and fine tuning of insulin requirements can be done without a hospital stay. Many diabetics manage quite well by consulting their doctors over the telephone between routine checkups. The most important part of therapy is that the diet and the insulin injection should be well coordinated. In most patients with Type II diabetes and gestational diabetes, however, insulin therapy can be initiated on an outpatient basis.

The most common side effect of insulin treatment is hypoglycemia. This usually occurs because of missed meals or snacks or erratic meal timing, excessive insulin dosage, or unplanned exercise. Other causes include failure to reduce insulin dosage after illness and after pregnancy, which require temporary periods of increased dosage, or failure to decrease insulin dosage after weight loss, which reduces insulin requirements. The symptoms of hypoglycemia are dizziness, impaired concentration, hunger, sweating, palpitation, seizures, and semicoma or coma. All patients on insulin therapy must be educated about the symptoms of hypoglycemia. Other side effects include insulin allergy, insulin-induced edema (swelling), lipoatrophy (wasting), and lipohypertrophy (growth).

Diabetes and Pregnancy

Normally in the first three months of pregnancy, nondiabetic women tend to have low levels of blood sugars, because maternal hormones (estrogen and progesterone) increase the action of insulin. But in the later half of pregnancy, women's insulin requirements increase; this happens because an insulin antagonist hormone from the placenta (human placental lactogen) produces relative insulin resistance. After a woman eats, resistance to the insulin action raises the levels of glucose and other nutrients and shunts a larger share of glucose and ammonia from the mother to the fetus. The fetus needs this greater share in the last half of pregnancy, which is the period of maximal fetal growth. In mothers with borderline B-cell function, these metabolic changes will result in gestational diabetes. *Gestational diabetes,* by definition, occurs during pregnancy and disappears after delivery. It should be noted that gestational diabetes often is a warning that diabetes may occur later in life. Pregnant women with preexisting diabetes need increased doses of insulin.

Fasting during pregnancy may cause production of a metabolic breakdown produce called ketone bodies in diabetic mothers, therefore omission of a single meal (for example, during a routine laboratory procedure or test) may have significant impact and could be dangerous, because ketone bodies have been said to be detrimental to the fetus.

If diabetes is poorly controlled during the first few weeks of pregnancy, the risks of spontaneous abortion and congenital malformation of the infant are increased. Later in the pregnancy, *polyhydramnios* (an accumulation of too much amniotic fluid) is also common in women with poorly controlled diabetes and may lead to early delivery. Fetal distress may develop in the third trimester of pregnancy if diabetic control is inadequate and careful fetal monitoring must be used to prevent stillbirths. The high incidence of *fetal macrosomia* (oversized fetus) has increased the risk of traumatic vaginal delivery, and primary cesarean deliveries are more common in these cases. Other neonatal risks can include respiratory distress syndrome, hypoglycemia, newborn jaundice, and poor feeding. However, some of these problems are limited to a few days, and childhood development is normal. Despite these complications, diabetic women now have a 97 percent to 98 percent chance of delivering a healthy child if they adhere to a program of careful management and surveillance. Accordingly, diabetic women are started on aggressive insulin therapy at the time of planning for a new infant.

Gestational diabetes occurs in 2 percent to 3 percent of pregnant women. It is caused by hormonal and metabolic changes. Once the diagnosis has been made, the woman should be placed on a diabetic diet, modified for pregnancy. Usually, blood sugar returns to normal after the delivery of the baby.

Now that people can measure blood sugar at home, patients can alter their dietary intake or insulin dose to maintain the blood glucose range.

The Diabetes Health Care Delivery Team

If you have diabetes, you may need several health experts, a team, to help you. The team consists of a physician, nurse educator, nutritionist, exercise physiologist, social worker/psychologist, pharmacist, and podiatrist. Your needs may vary, depending on the stage of the disease and according to your individual history, educational experience, coping mechanisms, and family or community support. The team's responsibilities fall into four sequential categories: medical management, education, support, and reevaluation.

The members of the diabetic health team and their responsibilities are summarized below.

Patient: provides basic information on the personal impact of the disease and therapy

Physician: assesses the physical and emotional status of the patient and initiates education and therapy

Registered nurse: focuses on education, implementation of therapy, assessment of skills, and their integration into life-style

Nutritionist (registered dietician): prescribes and implements a dietary plan based on individual needs

Exercise physiologist: monitors intensity duration, frequency, and results of specific exercise to meet the patient's needs

Social worker or psychologist: focuses on the impact of diabetes on a psychological or social level and helps to develop coping mechanisms that will lead to the acceptance and the social integration of the disease state

Podiatrist: provides preventive and therapeutic care of the feet

Ophthalmologist: provides preventive and therapeutic care of the eyes

Pharmacist: provides information about medication and instruction in the use of monitoring devices

Notice that the doctor plays a small role. In fact, the person with diabetes has the major role. That is why *patient education* is the most important part of the management. The education begins after the acute medical problem is over. Education is necessary not only for the newly diagnosed diabetic patients and their families but also for the patients with diabetes of any duration who may never have been properly educated about their disorder or who may not be aware of advances in diabetic management. The "curriculum" should include explanations of the nature of diabetes, its potential acute and chronic complications, and information on how these complications can be prevented, or at least recognized early and treated early. All patients should be made aware of community agencies that serve as resources for continuing education. Patients receiving hypoglycemic treatment (either insulin or oral hypoglycemic) should wear a medic alert bracelet or necklace that clearly states that insulin or oral sulfonylurea drug is being taken.

Diabetes can be controlled effectively, but it needs to be understood and aggressively confronted if it is to be managed.

About the Authors

Dr. José F. Caro has served as chair of the Department of Medicine at Thomas Jefferson University in Philadelphia since July 1991.

A recognized expert in the care and treatment of diabetes, Dr. Caro was program director of a major project from the National Institutes of Health (NIH) to study the mechanisms of insulin resistance in obesity and Type II diabetes. His work represents the first program in the world to investigate human tissue at the cellular level in the study of insulin resistance.

He has completed a fellowship in endocrinology and metabolism at the University of Rochester School of Medicine and Dentistry. He was both a fellow and a resident in internal medicine at Jefferson. He earned his medical degree at the School of Medicine in Madrid, Spain, and at Montevideo, Uruguay.

Dr. Caro is author or co-author of more than 160 scientific papers and abstracts, primarily on diabetes and related subjects.

Dr. Rishi Rastogi is a fellow of Dr. Caro and was training under him at the time of publication.

QUESTIONS FOR THE DOCTOR

Q: *I've been told my father has a disease called diabetes insipidus. Should he be eating a special diet?*

A: Although it shares the name diabetes, this disease is very different from diabetes mellitus, the subject of this chapter. People with *diabetes insipidus* urinate as much as three liters every day, and the urine that they make is very dilute. It does not have the concentration of normal urine. Diabetes insipidus is caused by many complicated factors, some of which are regulated by the brain, others by the kidneys. The danger of diabetes insipidus is that it can lead to dehydration. People try to keep up with the fluid they need by drinking excessive amounts. Diabetes insipidus can run in families, it can be acquired as a result of head trauma or neurosurgery, and it can also be caused by infections and even by a tumor. The key to the treatment of diabetes insipidus is finding the cause. Most doctors try to stabilize the patient while they search for this cause.

Q: *I am seventeen years old, and I'm tired of taking my insulin. I'm seriously considering stopping. My parents are frustrated with me. I'm frustrated with my disease.*

A: *Refusal* is very normal; in fact, medical books have chapters written about it. Many people your age do not want to think of themselves as having a serious disease and are frustrated by the limited actions imposed by an illness. You can take heart, however, because insulin allows you to control your diabetes and, in most respects, you are able to live a normal life. Remember that diabetes is a disease that causes damage over time, and uncontrolled diabetes can cause severe damage over time to the kidneys and to the nerves and to the blood vessels that lead to the heart. It is critical that you take your medication and control this damage, because down the road you will pay a heavy price if you don't. I know that you have to make many life-style changes, but believe me, all you have to do is see the ravages of uncontrolled diabetes in someone in their mid-thirties or early forties and you will realize how important it is to control the disease now. Good luck, and realize you are not alone in this problem.

Q: *What do you think about the new research in the treatment of diabetes?*

A: It is my understanding that the greatest research is actually being done in the treatment of Type I, the juvenile form of diabetes. Scientists are looking at the immunological causes of the disease. It is believed that somehow the islet cells of the pancreas are attacked by the body and that if there is some way to prevent islet cells from being destroyed, diabetes can be avoided. There are all sorts of theories about what causes diabetes, but at the present time the exact cause is not known. Exciting work is being done at several major medical institutions, including the University of Pennsylvania. This work is looking at the transplantation of islet cells in rats. The doctors have been able to take islet cells from a healthy rat and place them, not in the pancreas, but in the thymus gland of a diabetic rat. The diabetes has been reversed in the diabetic rat.

Why transplant the cells to the thymus? The biggest problem with transplantation of any organ is that the person who receives the transplant can reject the organ. That is why people who have had heart transplants and liver transplants have to take special medication to avoid the rejection. Islet cells are so small, however, that they can be transplanted almost anywhere. Doctors have found that if they transplant them into the thymus gland, it does not reject them. This has only been successful in rats, but this preliminary work shows promise.

The adult form of diabetes appears to have a genetic link. In fact, if one twin gets adult diabetes, the chances are 90 percent that the other twin will get it as well. Researchers are looking at genes that could cause this disease, and it is hoped that, as genetic technology improves in the coming decade, more can be done about diabetes. But remember, the adult form of diabetes can be controlled quite effectively through diet and exercise in a large number of cases.

Q: *My doctor has suggested laser surgery on my eye. Will this be painful?*

A: Well, there are many reasons why you may require laser surgery on your eye. I am assuming that you are referring to a change that is a result of diabetes. But, regardless of the cause, laser surgery is not painful while it is being done. All you perceive is the flashing of a light. I suggest that you talk to your ophthalmologist about the reason or reasons he or she feels that you need laser surgery, and then discuss your fears. Remember that, although laser surgery is often done in a doctor's office, it is still a surgical procedure. You may want to talk to one or more doctors about the best treatment for you.

While we are on the subject, the use of the laser has made remarkable changes possible in the treatment of *diabetic retinopathy*. Because of the laser, people who once may have been doomed to a loss of vision are able to live healthy, productive lives, without that disability.

Q: *If insulin is a cure for diabetes, why do groups like the American Diabetes Association continue to try to raise money?*

A: This is a common misconception. Insulin is not a cure. It is simply a form of treatment that helps buy time until a cure is found. The American Diabetes Association and others who work for the treatment of diabetes are focusing a great deal of their time on patient education and research. It is only through understanding their disease that diabetics will reduce their chances for long-term complications, and it is only through research that a cure will be found.

6

Exercise and Sports Medicine

Ray A. Moyer, M.D.

Sports and medicine have been intertwined since
Greco-Roman times, and physical activity has long been known to contribute to good health. Hippocrates wrote a chapter to athletes in training in which he stressed that eating by itself will not maintain well-being;
humans must also exercise. Galen's art of preserving health required vigorous activity, which was measured as an increased demand on the cardiac and respiratory systems. For over a thousand years, the basic tenets
of medicine were derived from Galen's six nonnaturals: air, food and
drink, motion and rest, sleep and wake, excretion and retention, and
the passions of the mind. The Industrial Revolution and urbanization
were associated with a national decline in health standards caused by too
much food, too much sleep, and too little exercise. At that time, an
effort was made to reestablish a self-help or self-regulation attitude to
reverse the trend. In the 1950s and 1960s, activity tests of military re-
cruits and school children demonstrated the poor physical status of the
American youth. In response to this, schools restructured physical education programs to improve the level of physical fitness in growing children;
at the same time, a national education program was instituted to encourage an increased level of activity in the adult population.

From the 1960s on, there has been a gradually increased awareness of
the need for regular activity in order to maintain physical and psychological health. Consequently, there has been a gradually increased participation in organized athletics and individual exercise programs. The

present-day enthusiasm for exercise and wellness, however, is just the latest flowering of a tradition dating back to Greco-Roman times. The association of fitness and appearance is a major driving force in following the exercise fad in present-day society, where mass communication places such a high premium on physical appearance. The highly visible and highly paid athlete is an obvious identity model for today's youth and represents an encouragement toward competition in athletics. Statistics show that about 25 percent of all females and about 50 percent of all males from ages eight to sixteen are engaged in competitive athletics. This represents a major increase over the past ten years. A similar increase has been evident in the number of adults participating in regular exercise programs.

What Is a Sports Injury?

Injuries that occur in athletes and other active individuals are not unique. The same anatomy is affected in a sprained ankle, regardless of how it occurs and regardless of a person's vocation or avocation. Athletes define a sports injury in terms of their own preinjury level of conditioning and their postinjury functional expectations. Sports medicine is concerned with injuries that prevent or limit participation in athletic activities. The physician gives appropriate care for the injury but also gives advice and direction to enable the patient to maintain overall strength and cardiovascular conditioning while he or she is recovering. The physician monitors rehabilitation and an accelerated or decelerated exercise program, depending on the patient's response to treatment. The athlete should be able to perform all required activities in the sport before resuming unlimited competition. The objective of treatment is to return the athlete to his or her preinjury functional level as quickly and as safely as possible. The success of treatment is measured by resumption of activity without reinjury.

What Is Sports Medicine?

Over the past twenty years, sports medicine has developed into a structured discipline of broad dimensions. Through the efforts of individuals in medicine, biomechanics, exercise physiology, nutrition, pharmacology, and physical and athletic training, programs for the treatment and prevention of injury and fitness programs for the young and old have been more definitively outlined. Analysis and continued modification of these programs should result in better health standards. One of the major activities in sports medicine is the development of coordinated programs to enable an individual to achieve a desired level of fitness (a conditioning program) and to help an injured individual stay fit while recovering (a rehabilitation program).

The component parts of conditioning and rehabilitation programs are the same; they include strength, flexibility, cardiovascular conditioning, and agility or sports-specific exercises. Conditioning and rehabilitation differ with regard to starting points, ultimate goals, and the intensity of exercise in the pursuit of those goals.

Conditioning

A conditioning program begins with healthy individuals whose aim is to increase their present functional capacity. Cardiac function is the main limiting factor in endurance activity. The threshold of activity needed to benefit from *cardiovascular training* is an effort that will raise the heart rate to approximately 70 percent of one's maximum heart rate. (To determine the maximum heart rate, subtract the individual's age from 220.) Cardiovascular conditioning targets the lungs, where oxygen is taken in, the heart vasculature, for the delivery of oxygen around the body, and the muscles' ability to use the oxygen that is delivered. Improved cardiovascular conditioning requires that between thirty minutes and sixty minutes of activity be done three to four times a week, with the heart beat raised to between 60 percent and 75 percent of one's maximum heart rate.

The basic strategy to improve an individual's strength is *muscular overload*. There are multiple programs designed to improve strength, but the aim of each program is to work the muscles to their highest level. There are three different types of strengthening exercises: Isometric exercises use static muscle contractions in which the muscle is flexed as hard as possible, but without motion. Isotonic exercises consist of moving a fixed amount of weight through a range of motion. This is the most common type of strengthening exercise performed. Isokinetic exercises require specific equipment, which is expensive, but allow the muscle to be worked maximally at every point through the range of motion. All three modes of exercises can demonstrate increased strength if they are done appropriately.

The use of *flexibility exercises* has been associated with a reduction in muscle strains or pulled muscles in competitive athletics. The higher the level of activity, the more the flexibility exercises are needed. Flexibility exercises are best done after a warm-up, which allows for an increase in body temperature that makes the muscles and tendons more pliable and more easily stretchable, increasing the effectiveness of the exercises. After a warm-up, the muscles should be stretched five to thirty seconds, maintaining a constant tension, and then be allowed to relax. Ten repetitions are adequate. Flexibility exercises should be done statically, not ballistically or in a bounding fashion. A bouncing-type stretch only causes a reflex contraction of the musculature and does nothing to improve one's overall flexibility. Flexibility exercises done against muscular contraction is termed *proprioceptive neuromuscular facilitation* (PNF), and these are thought to be the most effective type of flexibility exercises. After injury, PNF stretch is helpful in preventing recurrence.

The final component of a conditioning program are *agility exercises* or *activity-specific exercises*. These include: jumping drills, throwing drills, and agility drills. Sports-specific exercises help improve coordination in the execution of a sport. Many times these drills are defined by the coach or the athletic trainer.

The adage "No pain, no gain" has raised questions; nevertheless, conditioning requires a level of effort that causes some tissue breakdown, subsequent soreness, and, possibly, pain. As yet, there is no good explanation for the delayed onset of muscle soreness that commonly occurs one to three days after an increase in a person's normal activity. The only way known to prevent or resolve the soreness is to go through the conditioning program and to finally reach the level of training appropriate for the desired level of performance. A critical aspect of conditioning is that one must allow sufficient time to reach that level of activity so that the program does not result in injury. Even in the absence of injury, however, some soreness will occur.

Rehabilitation

Whereas the conditioning program takes a healthy individual to a higher level of functional performance, in rehabilitation, an unhealthy individual is working to regain his or her normal level of activity. During rehabilitation, the adage "No pain, no gain" is inappropriate. The individual must accommodate the intensity of the exercises to his or her tolerance during rehabilitation.

In rehabilitation, the severity of the individual's injury dictates the

initial treatment and rehabilitation plan. Injuries commonly cause localized swelling, associated with pain, decreased motion, and reflex inhibi-
tion of muscular activity. The initial treatment is aimed at controlling
pain and swelling; this includes rest, ice, compression, and elevation
(RICE). Following acute care, the first objective of rehabilitation is to
regain a full range of painless, fluid motion. Until comfortable motion is
reestablished, strengthening exercises should be minimized or avoided.

Initially, isometric strengthening execises are done, because they are
the easiest. The goal is to help maintain, or at least to minimize, the
potential for muscular atrophy. If exercises are too painful or too difficult,
a muscle stimulator may be used temporarily to maintain some muscle
tone. When motion is restored and swelling is controlled, more aggressive strengthening exercises can be done with free weights or with weight
machines. Increases in the weight used must occur gradually to avoid
an overuse or overstress injury, which can result in a setback. During
rehabilitation, strengthening exercises should be done two to four times
a day. When strength has been restored, a maintenance or conditioning
and strengthening program requires exercises only three to four times a
week. The mode of cardiovascular conditioning depends on the severity
of the injury and the anatomy involved. Cardiovascular exercises include
pool exercises, walking, bicycling, and, finally, running. The mode and
intensity of exercise is advanced to patient tolerance. Restoration of body
function to preinjury level during rehabilitation requires patience, direction, and attention to the body's reactions.

Sports Injuries

Injuries that occur as a result of sports activities are divided into two
groups: overuse, or stress, injuries and acute injuries, secondary to direct
or indirect trauma.

Overuse Injuries

Overuse injuries have familiar names, such as shinsplints, tennis elbow, tendinitis, jumper's knee, and stress fracture. Because overactivity
or overuse is a major contributing factor in the development of these
kinds of injuries, their treatment necessarily requires a reduction, to some
degree, in the offending activity. Although the last thing athletes want
to hear is a doctor's recommendation to stop their sports activity, for

most stress injuries some reduction in activity is needed, even though they need not stop entirely.

With any exercise, stress is associated with how often, how long, or how hard somebody is pursuing a given activity. Reduction in stress means a decrease in one, two, or all three of these stress areas. For example, in running, it may mean running slower, going shorter distances, or not running on hills. A thrower might have to throw with less velocity, less often, or for shorter distances. For swimmers it may mean changing strokes, going shorter distances, or swimming at slower speeds. Changes in these stress factors are termed "relative rest." Total rest is sometimes needed to allow resolution of an overuse injury, but total inactivity leads to muscle atrophy, overall deconditioning, and further weakness. Consequently, returning to previous levels of performance is more difficult. Relative weakness is, in part, the cause of overuse injury. A return to a preinjury level of activity requires that the injured part heal stronger than it was when the injury first occurred.

The treatment of overuse injuries requires relative rest, plus a rehabilitative exercise program. The exercises are not nearly as stressful as the offending activity. The essence of rehabilitation is submaximal strengthening and adequate stretching exercises, which stimulate healing processes to make the injured part stronger and less susceptible to recurrent injury when returning to competitive sports. This is what could be termed the "callous effect." It is analogous to a situation in which an individual gets blisters from gardening for three hours straight after having been inactive all winter or from playing three sets of tennis without having prepared adequately. If these activities were done in short repetitive bouts, over a two-week period, the skin's response would be to form a callous. Calloused skin is stronger and better capable of tolerating excessive pressure. The same concept is applicable to overuse injuries of the musculoskeletal system. When a person with a stress injury does an exercise regimen of minimal stress and many repetitions, his or her injured area will "form a callous," so to speak, and become stronger. Performing prescribed exercises and using relative rest in the treatment of overuse injuries may seen boring and too easy, but they are both essential for successful treatment.

Everybody wants to win at sports. The willingness to prepare often spells the difference between success and failure in competition. The second step in the care of overuse injuries is preparedness, which means going through rehabilitation; but, the first step is preventing them, which means engaging in an appropriate preactivity conditioning program.

Heat Injuries and Fluid Replacement

During periods of extreme muscular exertion, well-conditioned athletes are at risk for heat injuries. The three types progress from heat cramps, the mildest form, to heat exhaustion, and finally to heat stroke, the most severe. *Heat cramps,* commonly in the leg or abdomen, may also be associated with dizziness, lethargy, and nausea. These mild heat problems can be readily resolved by moving the affected individual to a cool area, applying cool towels, providing shelter from the sun, and giving fluids. The critical factor is fluid replacement. At every stage of heat injury, the primary problem is fluid depletion, which results in a lowered blood volume. Fluids can be replaced in the form of water or electrolytic solutions. The injured person obviously needs to drink the appropriate fluids, but he or she may not be able to take in a sufficient quantity quickly enough. During competition, athletes may lose eight to ten pounds, the equivalent of four to five quarts of water. It is almost impossible for someone to drink this much fluid in a short period of time, but three quarts of intravenous fluid can be administered easily within a half-hour to forty-five minutes and will readily correct a state of dehydration. The treatment must take place promptly to prevent the progression of heat cramps to a more severe stage.

Heat exhaustion is characterized by unsteadiness to the point of collapse, and lethargy and confusion to the point of unconsciousness. Breathing is rapid and shallow; the heart rate also is rapid but the blood pressure is adequate for perfusion of the heart, kidneys, and skin. The individual is still sweating, and this is a critical factor. Body temperature is elevated but this is not as important as the individual's ability to dissipate internal heat, primarily through evaporation of sweat.

The major worry with heat injuries is that there is not always a smooth, gradual progression from the mild form of heat cramps to the potentially catastrophic state of heat stroke. A common misunderstanding is that these injuries occur in the poorly conditioned athlete. On the contrary, it is the highly conditioned athletes that can push themselves to the extremes of muscular exertion, where the dangers of severe heat injuries exist. The highly conditioned athlete who has pushed himself or herself to the state of exhaustion requires prompt treatment.

Heat stroke occurs when a person has become so dehydrated that he or she ceases sweating; the body temperature rises precipitiously to temperatures up to 107 degrees, which can cause irreversible muscle and central nervous system injury. The temperature of the athlete is an important factor in determining whether heat stroke will cause permanent injury, but it can be misleading in assessing potential damage. Temperatures in the low hundreds can give a false sense of security. Oral temperatures are worthless in evaluation, and athletes have suffered heat stroke and died with recorded rectal temperatures as low as 102 degrees. Because there is not necessarily a gradual progression from heat cramps to heat stroke, even a highly conditioned athlete may move very rapidly from a state of exhaustion to a catastrophic level of heat stroke. Even the mildest forms of heat injuries, therefore, must be treated promptly and aggressively.

Ten to fifteen years ago, salt tablets were a part of the treatment of heat injury. Salt tablets are unnecessary and may do some harm. Oral intake of salt increases the salt concentration in urine and sweat; there, salt can act like a sponge and may increase fluid loss through sweating and urination. If dietary salt is restricted, the kidneys and sweat glands limit salt loss through these excretions and maintain an appropriate circulating electrolyte balance.

Prevention measures against heat injuries should be part of all sports activities. Fluids should be made readily available during practice and competition. Athletes in training should have regular weight checks, and if weight loss is continuous over several days, it is necessary to restrict their activities to allow for adequate rehydration and weight stabilization. Environmental conditions are also important. When the temperature and humidity index combined equal 160 degrees, practices should be reduced or changed to cooler times. Competitive athletes often play in severe conditions and must train to develop tolerance for environmentally extreme factors. *Acclimatization* training takes two to three weeks, and practice schedules should be planned if severe playing conditions are expected.

Children and Sports Injuries

Physical activity is as important in childhood as it is in adulthood, because children's activity patterns tend to be continued into adult life. Prior to puberty, boys and girls experience parallel strength gains with exercise. Once the male hormones become active, strength gains accelerate in boys and surpass those possible in girls. Before puberty, strength gains with exercise are not remarkable, but regular exercise can be beneficial and has not been associated with any significant musculoskeletal injury. Endurance exercises probably would improve cardiovascular conditioning in children, but few children are interested in the types of activities needed to see these gains.

Growing children present unique problems as regards sports injuries because of the potential injury to the growth plate (or *epiphyseal plate*). The growth plate is specialized cartilage found at the ends of arm and leg bones which provides for growth in length or height. Although the growth plate is the weakest part of the growing skeleton, it is the site of less than 20 percent of orthopedic injuries in children. Still, physicians, coaches, and parents must be alert to possible growth-plate injuries, whose complications can result in limb-length differences or limb misalignment. Preadolescent boys and girls actually have a lower injury incidence than do adults. It is in adolescence, when children become heavier, stronger, and more physically coordinated, that an abrupt rise in injuries occurs.

Overuse or overstress injuries may affect the growth plate. For example, *Osgood-Schlatter's disease*, a commonly recognized injury, affects the proximal growth plate of the tibia, at the knee. It rarely causes any long-term disability, and in most cases, the only evidence of it in adulthood is a boney prominence just below the kneecap. Fifteen to twenty years ago, *little leaguer's elbow* was a common malady. This injury to the growth plate of the elbow occurred as a result of overuse or abuse in the throwing athlete. The mildest form of little leaguer's elbow is an inflamed joint. With rest, which may require months, normal elbow function can be regained. If the disease process is allowed to progress, it can result in bone chips, loss of motion, and permanent functional limitation. Rule changes and appropriate restrictions in pitching during little league games has almost eliminated this injury. Currently, it seems more common in gymnasts.

Over the past ten years, increasingly, young swimmers have achieved elite performance levels as a result of high-powered swimming programs for preadolescents and the ability of athletes to push through the rigors of training. Swimming programs have been developed by champion coaches to develop champion swimmers. However, only a small percentage of swimmers have the physical strength or physical activity to reach the elite level. The worry is that some athletes will be pushed, to their own detriment. The shoulder is maximally stressed with the lifting and swimming training schedule. The "no pain, no gain" attitude may cause chronically sore shoulders in young swimmers, which may compromise their swimming during their competitive years and which may continue to be symptomatic into adulthood. Parents should be aware of the potentially serious nature of shoulder complaints and should be satisfied that the child's program is taking the precautions needed to avoid irreversible injury.

Coaches of children have a significant job. They must not only be encouraging and enthusiastic but must also maintain an awareness that growing children do not have the physical or psychological strength to measure up to the standards of the college or professional athlete; these are inappropriate goals for them. Children mature at different ages, experience different periods of awkwardness, and develop skills at different rates. Coaches of preteens must concentrate on keeping the youths active in sports by nurturing skills and encouraging effort, not by focusing solely on deficiencies. Coaches can have a major influence on a child's attitude toward sports, but parents have the ultimate responsibility to make sure that the appropriate goals are pursued.

The Aging Athlete

Physical changes of age are obvious and inevitable. The aging process causes a decrease of muscle mass, an increase in the percentage of body fat, a decrease in bone mineral, and a decrease in cardiovascular conditioning. Despite their inevitability, these effects can all be reduced or slowed by a regular exercise program. A person's strength peaks around age thirty. Thereafter, it may plateau or regress up to age fifty, depending on conditioning efforts. After age fifty, despite training, cardiovascular conditioning and strength decline. With effort, they can be maintained to within 80 percent of one's maximum conditioning, even in the seventh decade. If a middle-aged individual has been sedentary for an extended period of time, training efforts can effectively improve strength and endurance. The threshold needed to see a cardiovascular effect requires thirty to sixty minutes of activity done three times a week, with enough stress to reach 60 percent to 70 percent of one's maximum cardiac rate. Strength improvements require a muscular contraction equivalent to about 70 percent of maximum, with seven to ten repetitions on a regular basis.

Activity is necessary to maintain or improve conditioning, but overuse of muscles may result in injury. One reason for susceptibility to injury in middle age is the gradual decline in strength and cardiovascular conditioning, which necessarily limits one's overall physical capabilities. Many weekend athletes have the mentality of youth and try to play as they once did, even though their physical peak has passed; and they often play with inadequate preactivity preparation. Participation in physical activities should never be discouraged because less participation contributes to the natural decline in physical conditioning. The middle-aged athlete needs more preparation to participate in competitive sports and more postactivity recovery time to allow for recovery from tissue breakdown and replenishment of energy and fluids. Overtraining or overexertion will result in musculoskeletal fatigue injuries. Fatigue also causes secondary suppression of the immune system, which makes the athlete more susceptible to common viral illnesses such as the common cold.

Improving Sports Safety Rules and Equipment

The evolution of equipment and rule changes in American football illustrates the efforts to improve safety in sports. In the early 1900s, a presidential commission, headed by Theodore Roosevelt, saved the game of football by outlawing the flying wedge, a tactical maneuver that had caused an alarming number of injuries and fatalities. In the 1930s, head gear was developed, and the gradual improvement in the quality of helmets reduced the number of head injuries. However, as the head became better protected, it became an effective point of attack. It came to be used as a battering ram in blocking and tackling, resulting in an increased number of severe neck injuries. Rule changes in the mid-1970s, outlawing this "spearing" technique, have significantly reduced the number of serious head and neck injuries in tackle football.

Among the controversies over equipment is that of the present status of knee braces. Many types of knee braces are available, but none has proved clearly superior. A lateral hinge brace is commonly seen on offensive and defensive football linemen, but it has not been demonstrated that it offers sufficient protection to be made mandatory. Parents or coaches, then, should not be thought negligent if players are not using knee braces in contact sports. Some believe that the main benefit of any brace is that it provides more sensory information to the central nervous system from the protected joint; in this way it allows the musculature to react more quickly and more efficiently to actively protect the joint. If this is true, a rubber sleeve can be of benefit. Postinjury, athletes usually can return to their preinjury level of activity more comfortably and quickly when they are braced or taped. Knee braces and taping the knee do not cause weakness of the knee joint, but players who require extreme agility often find that any type of knee support is too restrictive and taping is, therefore, considered undesirable.

The use of ankle taping and ankle braces has been statistically shown to reduce the frequency of ankle sprains. As in the knee, supports about the ankle do not weaken the joint or the supporting musculature. But they may effectively reduce the person's overall agility, and in some sports, such as soccer, this is unacceptable. Following injury, ankle supports provide protection, which usually allows the athlete to return to a higher level of activity more quickly, more comfortably, and more safely than would be possible without the supports.

Protection of the face and eyes is needed in many sports. Prior to the 1970s, despite the obvious benefit of face masks for ice hockey goal tenders, masks were never used. It took the courage and leadership of an all-pro player to break a tradition. Today, a face mask is a standard part of a hockey goalie's equipment. Goggles should be used in squash and racquetball; they are readily available but not used enough. Shields in little league baseball, a recent development, seem to be readily accepted by the players.

In recent years, a lot of attention has been focused on athletic shoes. Athletic shoes do not vary much within categories. Many brands provide adequate support and shock absorption. Basically, the individual needs to feel comfortable in the shoe. Adapting to new shoes is the same as adapting to different running surfaces. A period of time is necessary to allow for the shoe to be broken in, to avoid potential stress injury of the foot, ankle, or knee. In the early 1970s, data proved that shoes with long cleats used on grass and turf predisposed athletes to more knee and ankle injuries and led to a change in shoe design. The soccer-style shoe, with multiple short cleats, has become the standard.

Arguments are still waged over the benefits of natural surfaces versus artificial playing surfaces. To be sure, economics figures in the decision. Perhaps when the financial issues are resolved, the decision will be less biased and the selection of one over the other will be based on objective evidence.

Changes are often resisted, and constant evaluation of game and practice conditions are necessary to allow for objective decisions to justify the changes. Constant reevaluation of conditioning programs has improved training regimens, which has enhanced the player's ability to participate. Athletes must be mindful of all changes and make sure they register their impressions about whether changes in rules, equipment, or conditioning programs improve the quality and safety in their chosen sport.

The Sports Medicine Physician: Advocate for the Athlete

The first requisite of a sports doctor is to be a caring physician. Regardless of specialty training, all physicians start with the Hippocratic oath and with the objective to relieve pain and heal the injured. Because most sports injuries involve the musculoskeletal system, the majority of sports medicine physicians are orthopedists. However, injury may affect any organ system, and emergency care must be provided for the total possible spectrum of injuries. A sports physician plays a major part in total patient care. When other specialties are involved, the sports doctor or team physician may become a bridge of communication between the treating physician, coaching staff, parents, and the injured athlete. The sports doctor certainly must be part of the final decision-making process to determine when the athlete has satisfactorily regained adequate conditioning to return to his or her preinjury level of competition.

The objective of the sports physician is to return the injured athlete to competition as quickly and as safely as possible, with the least risk of recurrent injury. This requires an accurate diagnosis, in order to provide appropriate acute care, outline the optimal rehabilitation program, and render a reasonable prognosis for the time frame in which the desired goal may be realized. Athletes are often under pressure from many directions to resume competition. At the professional level, pressure may come from management, coaches, and fellow players. At the interscholastic level, it may be from coaches, parents, peers, and from the athletes themselves.

All injuries are potentially serious problems. The physician is responsible for evaluating and treating each injury as critically and as carefully as possible. The greatest failure of that responsibility occurs when a physician (or trainer) underdiagnoses or undertreats a complaint, or assumes, at any time, that the athlete's complaint is either exaggerated or psychosomatic. The physician must use all information available, including the player's symptoms, the doctor's own examination, the coach's assessment of the player's playing potential, and the trainer's evaluation of the athlete. A thorough examination may not always reveal immediately the exact cause of a player's disability. The lack of obvious pathology does not necessarily rule out injury or mean that pain is not present. In these instances, it may be necessary for the physician to resist suggestions that the player is malingering.

When outside pressures push athletes to participate beyond their capabilities, it is the physician's responsibility to support them against these pressures. When the physician's evaluation demonstrates an objective disability, which disallows safe participation despite an athlete's desire to play, the physician must then protect the athlete from himself or herself.

About the Author

Dr. Ray A. Moyer is an associate professor of orthopedics at Temple University School of Medicine and is director of the Center for Sports Medicine and Science at Temple University Hospital in Philadelphia, the first of its kind in the nation. Dr. Moyer heads a comprehensive program that includes treatment for sports injuries, education, and research activities. A leading orthopedic surgeon, Dr. Moyer is a graduate of the University of Pennsylvania Medical School. He completed an internship at the University of Vermont Medical Center and an orthopedic residency at Temple University Hospital.

Dr. Moyer also completed a three-year tour of duty as a flight surgeon in the U.S. Navy.

QUESTIONS FOR THE DOCTOR

Q: *Why is our country so exercise crazy?*
A: Obviously, there are many things that can contribute to this. Certainly, the media and their emphases on good looks and well-conditioned bodies has a lot do with our attitudes. But, there is more to it than that. At the time of the Industrial Revolution, human labor supplied 30 percent of the energy used by factories and farms in America. Since that time, this number has decreased to approximately 1 percent. People who do not do manual labor need another way to stay fit; they need another outlet. People who enjoy competition are now turning to exercise in larger numbers. For the most part, this is good. Remember, people in other countries get more exercise in the course of daily living than do Americans, and they may not need as much exercise.

Q: *Why is exercise so good at relieving stress?*
A: We don't really know. When someone is under stress, their body re-leases *epinephrine,* which can cause blood vessels to constrict and the heart rate to increase. Exercise creates similar effects. Among our ancestors, the original stress response was the "fight or flight" response. People's heart rates and epinephrine output increased in response to a danger, such as a ferocious animal on the attack. The stress response was very important because it allowed the individual to run and to escape more effectively. In the twentieth century, most of the time our stress is the result of such things as an aggressive boss or a near-miss collision on the highway. The same response that allowed our ancestors to run from danger still comes into play when we are under stress, but there is no purpose for the accelerated heartbeat or release of epinephrine. Those in the field of sports medi-cine believe that exercise serves as a satisfying way of creating and resolving a moderate stress response and is a valuable outlet that can be beneficial. But, remember, this is a theory, and there have not been sufficient studies to prove it.

Q: *What is the effect of exercise on blood lipids?*
A: There have been a great number of studies in this field. One study in particular, conducted on long-distance runners, found that the aver-age levels of high-density lipoproteins (HDL, the "good" cholesterol) were as much as nine points higher than in the control subjects. Run-ning and other forms of exercise have been shown to increase the good cholesterol. As few as five to ten miles of jogging each week can elevate a person's HDL. Running is not the only exercise that can accomplish this: Swimming, tennis, brisk walking, and soccer all serve the same purpose. They allow the heart rate to be increased so that the cardiovascular system is sufficiently taxed.

Q: *Is it possible to compare one form of exercise with another in their effects on the basal metabolic rate?*
A: Yes, it is. This can be quite interesting. There are charts that show a breakdown of virtually any form of exercise, but I will mention only a few. Desk work expends one and one-half to two mets. (One met is the energy expenditure at rest, equivalent to approximately 3.5 millili-ters of oxygen per kilogram body weight per minute). Think of a met as a unit of comparison. Here are some examples: If you were to repair the radio in your car, it would take two to three mets. Driving a tractor trailer in traffic takes three to four mets. Doing light carpentry takes four to five mets, but digging in the garden may use five to six mets. If you decided to dig a ditch instead of digging in the garden,

you would use seven to eight mets, and if you want out to shovel snow in the peak of winter, you would use more than ten mets. Now, you may realize why so many heart attacks occur when people are shoveling snow.

Let's look at this from a recreational standpoint. If you were to sit and play cards, you would use one and one-half mets. Golfing with a golf cart would take two to three mets, but if you pull your own bag cart, you would use three to four mets. A golfer who carries his or her own clubs uses four to five mets. That is the same amount that a person would use playing doubles tennis. A game of singles tennis uses an average of six to seven mets, which is the same amount one would use if one walked five miles per hour or cycled at eleven miles per hour. Playing a vigorous game of basketball can use eight to nine mets, and playing competitive squash can use more than ten mets. Obviously, these numbers can all change, depending on how vigorously and aggressively you perform the exercise.

Q: *Is it possible to get a rash while playing sports?*
A: There is a phenomenon called *exercise-induced anaphylaxis*. People who get this may have one occurrence or may suffer numerous episodes. Usually, it begins after moderate to intense exercise, with a feeling of fatigue, warmth, and perhaps itching throughout the body. In the next phase, red, raised welts, similar to those you would see in a drug allergy, appear. Full-blown attacks can happen next, causing choking, with respiratory distress, abdominal colic, as well as nausea and lightheadedness. A person may experience wheezing and headaches persisting for as much as four hours after the attack. No one seems to know what causes exercise-induced anaphylaxis, but studies have shown that the levels of histamine commonly found in other forms of allergy attacks are elevated in these cases. People who suffer from exercise-induced anaphylaxis usually recover quite well. There are no reported cases of life-threatening swelling of the larynx. Most people are able to return to an active exercise program.

7

Eye Conditions and Disease

David J. Ludwick, M.D.

Eye problems are very common. Even ordinary vision problems can make the most simple task a challenge. Among the most prevalent conditions are nearsightedness and farsightedness, which are caused by problems with focusing the light entering the eye. If the light is not focused exactly on the retina (the sensory membrane that lines the eye), a blurred image occurs, similar to a blurred photograph, obtained because your camera was not in focus. The further the light is focused away from the retina, the more blurred the vision.

Nearsightedness (myopia)—the inability to see distant objects clearly—is caused by the eye focusing the entering light in front of the retina, usually because the eye is slightly longer than normal. It can be treated by wearing glasses or contact lenses to refocus the light rays by pushing them backwards onto the retina.

Farsightedness (hyperopia)—the inability to see close objects clearly—is caused by the eye focusing the entering light behind the retina, usually because the eye is too short. Farsightedness is also treated by wearing glasses or contact lenses to pull the light image forward onto the retina. Young farsighted people can frequently overcome this problem because they can change the shape of the flexible lens inside their eyes. As far-sighted people get older (usually by their forties), however, their lenses becomes stiffer and these people are unable to change the lens shape. This is why farsighted people frequently begin to need glasses by the time they have reached middle age.

101

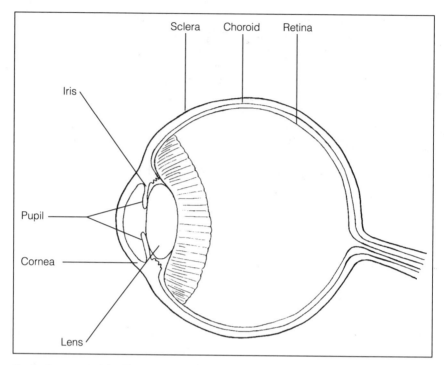

Basic Anatomy of the Eye

Astigmatism is due to an abnormal curvature of the cornea, which is the "clear window" on the front surface of the eye located in front of the iris. With astigmatism, the cornea is shaped like a football rather than a basketball. This causes the light to be focused differently, depending on which part of the cornea it enters, resulting in the distortion of images, which may appear elongated or slanted. Astigmatism is also treated by wearing glasses or contact lenses. They correct vision by making sure that all light is imaged on the retina.

As we get older, we increasingly face the frustrating problem of needing glasses to read. This phenomenon is called *presbyopia*. It has been called the "short arm syndrome" because to see clearly we need to hold reading materials farther and farther away. Presbyopia occurs in everybody, but it may not affect nearsighted people as severely as farsighted people. It is caused by the loss of lens flexibility due to aging. The lens needs to change shape to help focus on near objects. By our middle forties, however, the lens becomes less flexible and is unable to adequately change its shape. Reading glasses are usually prescribed to solve people's focusing difficulties. The lenses of the eyes continue to get stiffer as we age; therefore, the prescription strength of reading glasses frequently needs to be increased as we get older.

There is no reason to suffer from poor vision. For decades now, contact lenses have made life without glasses possible. There are several different types of contact lenses. Soft contact lenses are the most popular because they are comfortable and because people seem to be able to adjust to them more easily when they are first learning to wear lenses. Soft contact lenses come in three forms: daily wear, extended wear, and disposable. As the name suggests, *daily wear soft contact lenses* are removed at the end of each day. They are cleaned and sterilized so that they may be reworn the next day. *Extended-wear soft contact lenses* can be worn twenty-four hours a day, for two weeks to three months, after which they are cleaned and sterilized. But because of the extended period they are used without cleaning and sterilizing, they have been associated with increased eye infections. The newest form of soft contact lenses are *disposable*. These lenses can be worn for twenty-four hours a day for up to two weeks. They are then discarded. Disposable lenses have the advantage of not having to be cleaned or sterilized, but they can treat only farsightedness and nearsightedness. Unlike the daily wear or the extended-wear soft contact lenses, they do not treat astigmatism.

Hard or *rigid gas permeable contact lenses* generally give the sharpest vision of any contact lens, but they are less comfortable to wear and take a longer adjustment period than do soft contact lenses. They can correct all types of refractive errors (problems with focusing) and are especially good for people with astigmatism. Hard or rigid gas permeable lenses must be removed every night and cleaned and should never be worn during sleep.

It is very important that you see your contact lens specialist if you develop any pain, redness, or blurred vision while wearing contact lenses. These symptoms may indicate the presence of a corneal infection, protein deposits on your contact lenses, or that your lenses are too tight. Also, you should be examined by your contact lens specialist every six to twelve months to ensure that the contact lenses are not causing any unwanted side effects.

Surgery can also correct vision difficulties. Radial keratotomy is a surgical procedure performed by an ophthalmologist to correct nearsightedness by placing multiple incisions in the cornea in a radial fashion (like spokes on a bicycle wheel) to flatten the shape of the cornea. The re-shaped cornea pushes the light image back onto the retina. (Remember that nearsighted people have images that are focused in front of the retina.)

Astigmatism can also be surgically treated using a procedure called *astigmatic keratotomy*. Small incisions in the cornea correct its irregular curvature. Surgical correction of farsightedness is currently being investigated, but it has not been as successful as the surgical correction for nearsightedness. In addition, the use of the *excimer laser* is under investigation to correct refractive errors. It is expected to be approved by the Food and Drug Administration (FDA) to treat nearsightedness by 1996. The excimer laser reshapes the cornea by removing its superficial surface, similar to a carpenter's tool reshaping a piece of wood.

Some vision problems are not apparent until they are discovered by an eye doctor's exam. *Glaucoma* is the leading cause of blindness in the United States, but people with this disease usually exhibit no symptoms of it (they are *asymptomatic*). It more commonly affects African Americans, the elderly, and immediate family members of people with open angle glaucoma. Glaucoma causes damage to the optic nerve, which is like a wire connecting the eye to the brain. If the nerve gets damaged by glaucoma, all of the information collected by the eye is not transmitted to the brain and, subsequently, vision is decreased. The most common form of decreased vision caused by glaucoma is the loss of side, or peripheral, vision. With the gradual progressive loss of your peripheral vision, you eventually develop *tunnel vision*. Tunnel vision can be simulated by looking through a small tube, such as the kind that holds paper towels. If glaucoma is not treated, progression to complete blindness may occur.

Because glaucoma is generally asymptomatic, it can go undetected until severe loss of vision has occurred. When this happens, it is irreversible. The key to prevention is early diagnosis and treatment, so it is important to have periodic eye examinations by an ophthalmologist.

There are several types of glaucoma. The most common type is called *open angle glaucoma*. The hallmark of open angle glaucoma is increased pressure within the eye (i.e., increased intraocular pressure, usually greater than 21mm/hg). The main problem in open angle glaucoma is blockage of the drainage of fluid out of the eye. The eye produces this fluid, called aqueous humor, to provide nutrients to the inner eye structures. The amount of fluid produced by the eye usually equals the amount that drains out of the eye. In open angle glaucoma, however, the drain is partially blocked. As less aqueous humor drains out, more pressure builds up in the eye. The increased intraocular pressure squeezes the blood vessels and the nerve fibers of the optic nerve, causing damage and loss of vision. Early diagnosis of open angle glaucoma can be made by an ophthalmologist by (1) reviewing your medical and family history; (2) checking your intraocular pressure to ensure that it is not greater than 21 mm/hg; (3) examining your optic nerve for damage; (4) examining the drain of your eye (gonioscopy); and (5) testing for loss of your peripheral vision by visual field testing.

The treatment of open angle glaucoma usually consists of using eyedrops and taking medication that causes either a decrease in the aqueous humor production or an increase in the outflow of fluid through the drain of the eye. If the medications are not effective in controlling the glaucoma, a laser treatment (argon laser trabeculoplasty) to unclog the drain may be performed. Furthermore, surgery (trabeculectomy) can be performed to create a new drain for the eye.

Another type of glaucoma is called *angle closure glaucoma,* caused by a sudden complete blockage of the drainage of the aqueous humor from the eye because the iris (the colored part of the eye) covers the drain. This results in a very sudden and dramatic rise in intraocular pressure to exceedingly high levels, which can result in severe damage to the optic nerve and subsequent loss of vision in just a few hours.

Angle closure glaucoma is an ocular emergency and should be treated by an ophthalmologist as soon as possible. The symptoms of angle closure glaucoma include severe eye pain, eye redness, headache, nausea or vomiting, halos around lights, blurred vision, and hardened eyeball. Luckily, this form of glaucoma is less common. It occurs more frequently in farsighted people. To treat angle closure glaucoma one must bring the intraocular pressure down with eyedrops or oral medication. To prevent further attacks, however, a hole in the iris must be made, either surgically or with a laser. This prevents the iris from blocking the drain.

There are many other forms of glaucoma, some of these are pigmentary glaucoma, low tension glaucoma, pseudoexfoliative glaucoma, traumatic glaucoma, congenital glaucoma, neovascular glaucoma, steroid-induced glaucoma, and inflammatory glaucoma.

Another major eye problem is *retinal detachment.* To fully understand a retinal detachment, you must understand the function of the retina. The retina is a very complex, multilayered structure that takes light images and converts them into electrical impulses, which are then sent to the brain. The brain processes this electrical information to create the perceived visual image. The retina acts like photographic film in a camera. If the film is damaged (a retinal tear or hole) or is poorly positioned (partially detached retina), a poor quality photo (decreased vision) or no photograph (blindness) will occur.

A retinal detachment is caused by three general mechanisms. The first is a tear or hole in the peripheral retina. This can occur in patients who are nearsighted or who have thinning of the peripheral retina following trauma to the eye (a condition called *lattice degeneration*). The tear or hole may either extend to a "giant tear" or act as an entrance site for eye fluids to enter the hole and get under the retina, causing it to become elevated or "detached." Retinal tears may occur when the vitreous in the back of the eye shrinks because of aging. As it shrinks, it pulls on the retina, possibly causing a tear.

The second form of retinal detachment, caused by a pulling of the retina, is called a *traction retinal detachment.* Scar tissue is created in the eye, which pulls on the retina when the scar tissue shrinks. This type of retinal detachment is usually associated with diabetes and sickle cell disease.

The third form of retinal detachment is usually caused by fluid developing under the retina, without having a tear or hole. This can be caused by tumors and by leakage from retinal vessels (Coats's disease).

The most common symptoms of a retinal detachment are (1) grayish-colored, floating wavy spots or circles in your vision, (2) flashes of lights, (3) blurry vision, (4) loss of part of your vision (such as being able to see only part of someone's face), and (5) the sensation that your vision is disappearing, similar to a curtain closing.

The treatment for a retinal detachment varies according to the cause. With a small retinal hole or tear, occasionally all that is needed is a laser or freezing treatment around the defect to "spot weld" the retina. If it is a larger retinal hole or tear, removal of the fluid from under the retina and placement of an encircling band (scleral buckle) around the eye may be required. An alternative form of treatment, pneumatic retinopery, is to inject gas into the eye to push the retina back into its proper position. If the detachment is because of a tumor, radiation therapy may be needed. A traction retinal detachment in diabetics frequently requires removal of the vitreous and scar tissue with placement of an encircling retinal band.

If a retinal detachment is repaired early, sight can be preserved. If it is not treated or is allowed to progress to a complete retinal detachment, blindness can occur. Careful examination of your retina by an ophthalmologist using dilating eyedrops can detect early retinal problems that can be treated before a severe retinal detachment occurs.

One final eye problem to consider is a leading cause of visual loss in people over age sixty-five. *Macular degeneration* is an age-related disease that affects a small area of the retina called the macula. Despite being such a small area, the macular region is responsible for our ability to discern fine details and read small print. Macular degeneration is an inherited disease that predominantly affects Caucasians, causing gradual destruction of the macula as the person gets older. It results in a loss of central vision, not peripheral vision. The amount of visual loss varies from a mild decrease in vision to severe central vision loss, resulting in an inability to drive a car or read. However, it is very important to understand that macular degeneration will *not* cause you to become totally blind.

The symptoms of macular degeneration include blurring of vision when reading, development of small blind spots when looking straight ahead, difficulty reading because the blind spot does not allow you to see all the letters of a word, and vertical lines that may appear wavy or distorted. Macular degeneration may be diagnosed by a detailed examination of the retina by an ophthalmologist. If degeneration is present, it can be followed for progression by the daily viewing of an Amsler grid chart, which can be obtained from your eye doctor. If progression does occur, laser treatment may be beneficial to treat abnormal blood vessels that can develop and cause swelling or hemorrhages of the macula. Low-vision aids are also available. These include magnifying lenses, large-print books, "talking books" on cassette tapes, telescopic lenses for distance vision, check-writing guides, and large-dial telephones.

About the Author

Dr. David J. Ludwick received his medical degree from Temple University School of Medicine. His postgraduate training includes an internal medicine residency at Abington Memorial Hospital, outside Philadelphia, and an ophthalmology residency at the University of Maryland in Baltimore. Dr. Ludwick is chair of the Department of Ophthamology at Mercer Medical Center in Trenton, New Jersey, and he is certified by both the American Board of Ophthalmology and the American Board of Internal Medicine. He is a partner in the practice of ophthalmology at Brown and Ludwick Eye Associates. Their offices are located in Newtown, Pennsylvania, and West Trenton, New Jersey.

QUESTIONS FOR THE DOCTOR

Q: *What is dry-eye syndrome?*
A: Dry-eye syndrome affects many people over age fifty-five. It is caused by a reduction in the tears made by the tear glands in the eyelids. These tear glands are different from the lacrimal glands that are responsible for emotional tearing (i.e., crying). Dry-eye syndrome does not mean that you cannot cry. The normal fluid that keeps your eyes moist throughout the day either evaporates quickly or is not made in adequate amounts. This results in several problems, including (1) intermittent blurred vision, especially when reading or in the evening, (2) scratchy and burning eyes, (3) red eyes, and (4) tearing.

The treatment of dry-eye syndrome is to place artificial teardrops in the eyes. It is important to treat this condition because severe dry eyes can lead to scarring of the cornea and a permanent decrease in vision. If the articifial tears are not adequate, further treatment may be precribed by your ophthalmologist.

Q: *What is conjunctivitis?*
A: *Conjunctivitis* is an inflammation of the thin skin covering the eyeball. The symptoms include red eyes, discharge, crusting and stickiness of the eyelashes, and possibly some swelling of the eyelids. There are several different types of conjunctivitis. *Infectious conjunctivitis* is frequently known as "pink eye" and may be caused by a bacterial infection or a viral infection. It frequently occurs at the same time as a cold. It may be very contagious and is usually treated with antibiotic eye drops. Even though antibiotics do not cure viral infections, they are frequently prescribed to prevent secondary infections of the eye. Cool compresses may also be used to help relieve irritation and eyelid swelling. It is very important that those with infectious conjunctivitis are careful not to spread the disease to anyone else. Transmission of this condition can be minimized by washing hands frequently, using separate towels, and by avoiding the sharing of make-up. Many children are kept home from school to prevent the spread of their infection to other school children.

Allergic conjunctivitis is most common in spring or fall, when pollens are abundant, but may occur at any time of the year. Allergic conjunctivitis is not infectious and, therefore, it not contagious. It is an allergic reaction to pollen, pets, dust, or some other allergenic substance. Symptoms include redness, itching, tearing, and eyelid swelling. It is usually treated with cool compresses and antihistamine eyedrops. Occasionally, oral antihistamines and steroid eyedrops are needed.

Toxic conjunctivitis is caused by a chemical irritation of the eyes, such as from smoke, pollution, soap, or other chemicals. This problem usually resolves itself after the chemical irritant is removed. However, if the eye has been accidentally splashed with a chemical, it should be rinsed immediately with large amounts of water, for at least fifteen minutes, and the person should be seen at once by an ophthalmologist. Chemical injury can cause permanent damage to the eye, especially if it is an acid (found in bleach and batteries) or an alkali (found in drain cleaners, cement, lime, and paint thinner solutions).

Q: *Can the eyelid become infected?*
A: Infection of the eyelid *(blepharitis)* is very common. It frequently is associated with several skin diseases, including seborrhea, psoriasis, and acne rosacea. Symptoms of blepharitis include redness of the eyelid margin, crusting of the eyelids, swelling of the eyelids, eye redness, irritation, tearing, and intermittent blurred vision. The symptoms are usually worse in the morning. Treatment consists of washing the eyelashes once or twice a day with a cotton ball dipped in diluted baby shampoo (five drops in a small glass of warm water). This usually cures the infection in one or two weeks. If the infection persists, the addition of a topical antibiotic or combination antibiotic-steroid ointment will usually be curative. However, once the condition is cured and treatment is stopped, blepharitis may recur, and chronic treatment with daily washing of the eyelids may be required to keep it under control. If you wear eye make-up, do not wear it while you have the infection, and replace it with new make-up to avoid reinfection.

A *stye* (hordeolum) is an infection of the oil glands or of a hair follicle within the eyelid. It is frequently caused by an infection of the eyelashes spreading to the oil glands of the eyelid. A stye presents as a red, swollen, frequently painful, bump on the eyelid. It usually resolves itself with warm compresses to the involved eyelid for ten minutes, four times a day. If the stye does not go away within a few days, contact your ophthalmologist, who may prescribe topical or oral antibiotics. Frequent washing of the eyelids may also be prescribed if there is associated blepharitis. If they are treated early, styes are easily cured. If they are left untreated, however, they may progress to become a chronic infection called a *chalazion.* Chalazions are treated in the same manner as styes, but they are sometimes resistant to treatment. If so, they must be surgically drained and removed.

Q: What should I do if my child's eyes are not straight?

A: This condition is called *strabismus,* and it is frequently an inherited trait. There are two major types of strabismus, paralytic and nonparalytic. Paralytic deviations of the eye are due to nerve muscle damage. *Paralytic strabismus* may be associated with serious medical diseases, such as brain tumors, intracranial aneurysms, thyroid disease, diabetes, myasthenia gravis, infections of the central nervous system, strokes, or birth injuries. *Nonparalytic strabismus* either is an inherited trait or is due to farsightedness and usually presents in childhood.

Strabismus can result from one or both eyes turning in (called cross-eyed or *esotropia*), turning out (called *exotropia*), or turning up (called *hypertropia*). The deviation of the eyes may occur intermittently, especially when fatigued, or may be present constantly. The complications of strabismus can include double vision, loss of three-dimensional vision, poor cosmetic appearance, and decreased vision (called *amblyopia* or "lazy eye"). Amblyopia is a serious, but reversible, problem in children with strabismus. Amblyopia is the brain's method of preventing double vision. To alleviate the confusion of double vision, the brain selects the clearest image from one eye and suppresses the image from the other eye, thereby preventing double vision. This condition is reversible if treated by age six or seven. Treatment includes patching of the nonamblyopic eye to force the lazy eye to work, which subsequently results in improved vision. Once amblyopia has been corrected, eyeglasses to correct for farsightedness may be prescribed or surgery on the muscles of the eye may be performed to straighten the eye and to improve the cosmetic appearance of the eyes. Strabismus and amblyopia are both treatable; therefore, early examination by an ophthalmologist is very important.

Q: What is a corneal abrasion?

A: *Corneal abrasions* are scratches on the surface of the cornea. They are usually caused by trauma to the eye, for example, from a tree branch or fingernail, or by foreign bodies becoming embedded in the cornea. Symptoms include pain, redness, blurred vision, and tearing. Corneal abrasions should be seen by an eye doctor to ensure that there is no infection or foreign body embedded in the cornea that has to be removed. Abrasions are usually treated with antibiotic eyedrops, but they may require patching of the eye and occasional oral pain medication.

Many times corneal abrasions and embedded corneal foreign bodies can be prevented by wearing protective eyewear. This is especially important if you are exposed to chemicals, sharp objects, flying particles, and high-speed tools at your home or workplace. Protective eyewear is also important to help avoid eye injuries while playing sports such as hockey, squash, and racquetball. The speed at which the ball or puck travels in these sports is so fast that if it hits the eye, it can cause severe eye injury or blindness.

Q: *What is a cataract?*

A: A *cataract* is a clouding of the lens in the eye, which is normally clear and transparent. The lens is a dynamic structure that continues to grow throughout one's life. This constant growth eventually causes everyone to develop cataracts, if they live long enough. Certain conditions may cause the development of cataracts earlier in life. Some of these conditions are diabetes, inflammation in the eye, eye trauma, certain medications (steroids and thorazine), congenital cataracts secondary to birth defects, and infections during pregnancy that affect the newborn baby (measles, rubella, syphilis).

When you have a cataract, light passes through the cloudy lens and becomes scattered and distorted, resulting in a fuzzy image on the retina. In addition to decreased vision, cataracts may also cause a star pattern to appear around lights (especially when driving at night), frequent eyeglass prescription changes, sensitivity to light, glare in bright lighting, decreased brightness of colors, and, occasionally, double vision.

When should a cataract be removed? This differs from person to person and depends on the severity of the symptoms and their effect on daily activities, work, life-style, and so on. If you are developing any change in vision or loss of vision, report it to your eye doctor. A complete examination will determine if you are developing a cataract. If the cataract is interfering with your daily activities, then it is probably time to remove it.

Cataract surgery is usually performed under local anesthesia. Frequently, the patient can go home after the operation is completed, without having to stay overnight in the hospital. The development of new microsurgical techniques has made cataract surgery very successful. Following the removal of the cloudy lens, a new artificial intraocular lens is usually implanted to help the eye focus. Other options to the intraocular lens include contact lenses or cataract glasses. In general, the intraocular lens is the most popular choice because it does not require cleaning like contact lenses, and it does not cause distortion like cataract glasses. However, there are certain eye conditions in which an intraocular lens is not desirable. Your ophthalmologist will help you decide which option is best for you.

Occasionally, following cataract surgery your vision may again become hazy because of the development of a cloudy lens membrane. If this does develop, your ophthalmologist may suggest laser surgery to create a small hole in the cloudy lens membrane to help restore your vision.

Q: *What is diabetic retinopathy?*
A: *Diabetes milletus* affects approximately ten million Americans. It is a disease characterized by high sugar levels in the blood because of the body's inability to properly use and store sugar. Diabetes can affect your vision in several ways, including (1) temporary blurring of vision due to fluctuations in the blood sugar level, (2) development of cataracts, (3) development of glaucoma, and (4) the development of diabetic retinopathy.

Diabetic retinopathy is characterized by the weakening of blood vessels that nourish the retina. This leads to deterioration of the retina. The retina is like the film in a camera. If you have damaged film in the camera, you will not take good pictures. The same is true for your eyes. If your retina is injured, you will not see well.

The damaged, weakened blood vessels leak blood or fluid, causing swelling of the retina. If this swelling occurs in the macula, the center portion of the retina responsible for fine reading vision, your vision can be significantly decreased. This is called *background diabetic retinopathy.* Occasionally, the swelling will resolve on its own. More commonly, however, treatment by an ophthalmologist will be required. With this treatment, first you have a flouroscein angiogram, by which photographs of the retinal blood vessels are obtained to determine the location of the leakage. The eye doctor treats the sites of blood vessel leakage with laser treatments to seal the leaks. Once the leakage has stopped, the retinal swelling usually resolves itself and the vision is improved.

In the more advanced stage, called *proliferative diabetic retinopathy,* blockage of retinal blood vessels can occur, causing permanent destruction of small areas of the retina. Additionally, new blood vessel growth on the retina or optic nerve may occur. These new blood vessels are very fragile and may rupture, resulting in bleeding into the vitreous (clear substance that fills the center of the eye). The blood in the vitreous blocks light entering the eye and can dramatically decrease vision. Furthermore, the new abnormal blood vessels can cause the formation of scar tissue. This scar tissue can tug on the retina, causing it to be pulled off from the back of the eye. This is called a *retinal detachment* and results in severe visual loss and eventual blindness if not treated.

Treatment of proliferative diabetic retinopathy usually requires extensive laser treatment to the retina to reduce abnormal vessel growth. If bleeding occurs despite laser treatment or if there is very severe proliferative diabetic retinopathy, then a surgical procedure called vitrectomy may be performed. In this procuedure, vitreous, blood, and scar tissue pulling on the retina are removed from the eye. Repair of a retinal detachment may be combined with vitrectomy surgery to help restore vision.

Early detection and treatment of diabetic retinopathy is the best defense against vision loss. It is important to be seen regularly by an opthalmologist once diabetes has been diagnosed. If you experience any type of vision problems, contact your doctor immediately.

8

Health Care Choices

Mike Magee, M.D.

Choosing health care has become a major source of anxiety in America today. There is so much at stake that touches you personally and affects your family security, economic survival, autonomy, and control. Health care services are both complex and interrelated; so choosing health care involves a series of integrated choices. Who will be your physician? When do you use a physician extender, such as a nurse practitioner or nurse midwife? Are you choosing a physician for yourself or for your family? What hospital will you use if you need one? Who do you want "calling the shots"? How much health care can you afford? Where do you begin? Because the answers to the preceding questions will affect the decision you make about any of the others, you have to separate the elements of each and then consider them together in order to come to an overall decision that works best for your situation. This chapter explores the major issues for the key decisions you need to make. It focuses on choosing your doctor, choosing your hospital and preparing for hospital care, and determining how you will pay for medical care.

Choosing Your Doctor

Times certainly have changed, but one major concept has remained the same: We want to be as healthy as we can be!

When I was a boy back in the 1950s, choosing a doctor was the major decision for the health consumer. My father was a physician, with an

114

office attached to the house. His patients had relatively simple choices because health insurance was not common in those days. His patients who could afford to pay paid in cash. Those who would not pay were given free care. Few patients exercised their own judgment about their health care needs or their right to participate in health care decisions. They trusted my father and doctors like him to make the right decisions for them. The doctor alone determined hospital choice, appropriate treatment, and when to fight and when to quit, and his decisions were explained to his patients. Today, health care problems, the medical knowledge most people have, the variety of options for treatment, and the costs of health care are quite different. Physicians expect patients to be involved in decision. In today's world, then, the choice of a doctor is a part of the picture rather than the entire picture.

It is always better to choose a doctor when you and your family are well rather than when you are ill, because you can investigate, ask questions, shop around, and make a decision without time restraints or anxiety about an illness competing for your attention. It is also important to recognize that this is a very personal and individual decision. Communication styles and the approaches of different physicians vary. Begin by visualizing the perfect doctor for your family: Is he or she young or old, male or female, outgoing or reserved, brilliantly intellectual or down to earth? What style makes you the most comfortable?

Now you need to spend some time shopping around. Your most important source of information is probably those people in your family, at work, or in community associations whose opinions you respect. They can provide you with their reactions to the physicians they know and tell you who they would recommend, addressing issues of competence as well as style and cost. Another source of information is the physician referral services sponsored by many hospitals. These services are supported by extensive data banks that include information about the doctor's sex, age, training, board certification, geographic office location, special interests, and even personal family data and practice philosophy.

Once you have narrowed a list of possibilities, the most important source of information is a personal visit. When you contact the office to ask for a get-acquainted visit, you should ask about the fee; sometimes these visits are available free or at a reduced rate. When you visit, be attentive to the physician's office setting and assess the physician and his or her support staff in terms of their approach to timeliness, orderliness, friendliness, openness, and flexibility. Do you feel comfortable there?

Remember, qualifications alone will not support the perfect choice. For a good match, you should like the doctor, because a poor doctor-patient relationship can ultimately affect your care.

Once you have identified and catalogued what you are looking for in a doctor, have shopped around, and have made several office visits to different doctors, how will you make a final decision? One approach is to create a chart listing the essential characteristics, so that you can rate them from one (lowest) to five (highest) and see who receives the top scores. You might include:

Physician reputation

Physician personality

Office location

Flexibility of office hours

Accepts your insurance

Friendly, helpful office staff

Reputation of affiliated hospital

Communication and education skills

Willingness to take time with patients

Trustworthiness

When you have compared the scores and think you have a winner, you have one or two further things to consider. Who are the doctor's partners and are their reputations and philosophies similar to those of the doctor you plan to choose? Remember that no one can be available 24 hours, 365 days. So, to some extent, your choice of your physician is a choice of the partners or associates as well. When you choose a primary care physician, you are also choosing his or her referral specialists. For example, which cardiologist would your physician choose if you had chest pain, which surgeon if you needed your gallbladder removed, or which orthopedic surgeon if your child broke an arm? When you choose a doctor, you are also choosing a network of other physicians, laboratory services, and hospitals. So, as much as possible, you should define this network first.

Finally, for many people, the choice of physician is no longer the first question. Issues of health care affordability have become primary. If economic issues narrow your options for health care, you need to address the issue of physician choice within the confines of your particular health plan.

Choosing a Hospital

Just as no two doctors are alike, no two hospitals are alike. Just as one physician might be perfect for the purpose of primary, preventive health care and another more appropriate for specialty intervention, hospital services may also differ along the same lines. Forty years ago, hospitals provided fewer services, patients' hospital stays were much longer, and the cost of care was fully reimbursed. Today, the hospital is a high-tech center for advanced forms of diagnosis and treatment of very ill patients. Simpler cases are handled on an outpatient basis; in fact, over 50 percent of all of the procedures now offered at hospitals are done on an outpatient basis. This trend will continue as hospitals are increasingly built with the patient customer's needs and cost effectiveness in mind.

The ideal hospital can provide a balance of humanistic care and scientific care twenty-four hours a day, administered by a highly skilled and cooperative team of doctors, nurses, and health care managers. Easy access, time efficiency, and visible signs of good communication suggest that an institution is well run and knows its business. Humanistic qualities should be easily visible on a walk through a health care institution: the way the place feels, the sense of pride on the faces of employees, the sense of orderliness and friendliness, the physical layout and signage, the size and furnishings of the room, and the attitude of the people delivering the care. Is patient information material available? Do people interact with you and try to help you through these sometimes confusing institutions? Is there a chapel visibly present? Is there a strong presence of volunteers? Do the doctors and nurses take time to interact with the patients and their families?

Pivotal to a hospital's success and reputation is the standard of its clinical staff, including doctors, nurses, and allied health personnel. For prospective patients, hospitals remain a buyer's market. That is, in most areas of the country, most patients have an opportunity to compare the reputations of two or more institutions and choose between them. As with physician choice, the best way to determine the quality of a hospital is to ask. The worst way to make a choice is to rely on yellow pages ads, television advertising, or billboards. Former hospital patients are generally willing to describe their experiences, good or bad. In addition, in many states, outcome data, including deaths, complications, the length of stay for different procedures, and the overall rating of various hospitals by procedures, are becoming readily available. These data are being reported with greater frequency in the general press and should be available to consumers. Finally, the choice of a hospital is a very reasonable topic to discuss with your physician.

Which should you choose first: the hospital or the doctor? The answer depends on how much the health care institutions in your community differ. If there clearly is a front-runner in both comprehensive clinical care and humanistic approaches, an institution that has dramatically better results within a significantly friendlier and more efficient environment, you may wish to begin your exploration with this hospital. If you do so, your next step is to obtain a listing of physicians on the medical staff from that hospital to help guide your choice of physicians or insurance. Many hospitals have physician referral services, which may help you to narrow the choice as well. If there is limited choice of hospitals or if the general opinion is that all hospitals in your community are pretty much equal, you may want to choose the doctor first. When you are closing in on your choice of a hospital, it's worthwhile to visit the areas where you are most likely to be at some time in the future, such as the emergency room, the obstetrics unit, the surgery waiting area, and outpatient laboratories. How are people treated in these areas, and how long do they have to wait? How clean are these areas? How would you feel about utilizing these areas at 8 A.M., 8 P.M., or 2 A.M.? Does this hospital instill confidence in you?

Before you make a choice, ask yourself the following questions:

Does the hospital offer the services that you and your family need?

Does the hospital have experience in the conditions that you and your family have?

Does the hospital provide follow-up services, such as home care and nursing homes?

Are operating-room services, laboratory, radiology, and emergency services available around the clock?

Does the hospital have a well-thought-out approach to pain management?

Does the hospital provide community education programs?

Does the hospital have a coordinated system for preadmission testing for surgery and other procedures?

What types of referral connections does the hospital have for procedures or services it does not provide?

Does the hospital have in place pastoral care and bereavement services and other forms of social and emotional support for patients and family members?

What is the reputation of the medical staff and the nursing staff at the hospital?

Preparing for a Hospital Stay

Many people do not adequately prepare for a hospital stay, whether it be an elective or emergency admission. Generally, hospital stays generate some fear and anxiety. This is normal. If you gain some knowledge of the hospital before you choose it, you will feel much more reassured. If your admission is elective, you probably will be given some written material that explains the procedure that you will be going through, rules for visitors and friends, and so on. This information allows you to prepare yourself and your family for what will take place.

The key to a smooth hospital stay is to ask questions. Your doctor and his or her office staff should be able to provide clear answers to questions not only about your treatment and care but also about payments. Most hospitals' billing departments designate individuals to answer your insurance questions prior to hospitalization. The more questions you can resolve before to visit, the less anxiety you will feel about the hospitalization.

You should always consider preparing *advance directives*, no matter what the reason for hospitalization, especially if you have a serious condition. Advance directives tell your health care providers about the care you wish to receive or not receive when you become unable to express your wishes. The approaches to advance directives vary from state to state and generally are handled under the categories of durable powers of attorney, health proxies, or living wills. Your physician or the admission department of your hospital should have information to assist you.

Another important step in preparing for your hospitalization is to be certain that your family has a list of your important documents and their locations, including your will, insurance papers, bank account numbers, and investment information. It is also useful to have personal bills paid in advance and to assign duties for key chores, such as caring for pets and plants, picking up your mail and newspapers, or arranging for children's care.

You can make your return to home a little easier by arranging beforehand for someone to bring you home from the hospital. Consider who this might be if you were discharged during the day, night, or weekend. If you live alone and are concerned about your care after discharge, you should speak to your hospital's social work services department before your admission; they will be able to help answer your questions about home health care or a visiting nurse.

It is best not to bring large amounts of money or valuables such as jewelry to the hospital; they might be more secure at home. You should bring secure and well-marked containers for hearing aids or dentures, since it is very easy to misplace or lose these items on hospital nightstands. If you wear glasses, a neckstrap or case can help you keep track of them during your stay. You should also bring the personal items that you think you may need and clothing that will ensure your comfort.

As you head off to the hospital, you should be able to visualize where you are going, what the environment will be like, and what will be the major checkpoints in your care and recovery, including a general timeline. If all of this information is clear in your mind, you are well prepared.

Handling the Cost of Medical Care

Health care costs have risen and the use of health care insurance has become more complicated; thus handling insurance reimbursement for medical care has almost become more of a challenge than receiving the care itself. Two issues are of major importance when it comes to the choice of health care: *accessibility* and *affordability.*

Access to health care involves a number of issues, including choice of physician, choice of hospital, the distance you must travel for services, and ease of receiving emergency care. As health care costs have risen, insurance companies have attempted to control these costs by controlling health care access, for example, by defining the panel of doctors and hospitals involved with a particular insurance program and by ensuring that, through a variety of different strategies, people do not overutilize health care. Insurance companies' cost-containment programs often include requirements for second opinions, precertifications of admissions to hospitals, and same-day admissions rather than admitting patients a day before surgery. Cost containment also can entail refusal to pay for certain tests or procedures. Law requires insurance companies to specifically explain these rules to the purchasers of health insurance. The regulations can be quite detailed and confusing, and it is worthwhile to discuss them with your employer, insurance agent, hospital billing department, or physician before purchasing health insurance. You also should review the insurance rules pertaining to a particular condition or long-term treatment before entering the hospital, so that you will know the extent of your financial obligation.

The second important issue regarding health care choice is affordability. Most health insurance policies require a deductible amount, usually paid at the beginning of each calendar year; for example, you are required to pay $1,000 of your health care bill before your insurance begins reimbursing you. Instead, or in addition, your policy might pay 80 percent of all charges, leaving you to pay the remaining 20 percent. Some people purchase secondary insurance to pay what the primary insurance does not. Evaluate the cost of such supplementary plans to determine whether they will offset your medical care costs over the long term.

Once you have determined what you can afford and what degree of access to health care is allowed under the insurance plan, you may want to ask customers who are currently using the plan whether they are satisfied with it. It can be very helpful to talk to friends or acquaintances who have used the company you are considering. How easy is it to fill out the necessary forms? How rapidly are payments made? How easy is it to get information or authorization from the company? Are your friends happy with their choices? Doing a little survey work before you choose a health insurance plan can give you a clearer picture of the relationship you may have in the future with the insurance company.

Before you choose your insurance plan, be sure that you understand the fine print. Read the policy carefully to understand what is covered and what is not. Become familiar with the language of your plan; for example, a traditional plan has deductibles and copayments (a small amount that you pay with each visit). If you enroll in a managed-care plan through your employer, you will need to find out what physicians belong to that plan, including primary care physicians and specialists such as surgeons or cardiologists. You must keep your family's special needs in mind, because insurance plans differ in their coverage for such things as prescriptions, infertility treatments, and preventive care, such as eye exams. Some plans even offer incentives for membership in health clubs or weight-loss programs. It is important to examine your plan's ability to support preventive medicine. Are regular checkups covered, including yearly Pap tests, mammograms, prostate cancer and colorectal cancer exams?

If you are over age sixty-five, apply for Medicare. Although eligibility begins at this age, coverage is not automatic. Contact your social security office for help in enrolling for this protection. If you are unable to afford health insurance, arrange for a visit with your hospital's social service department to discuss payment options.

Once you have chosen a health insurance plan and are enrolled, there are steps that you can take to help protect you and your family and to prevent the future need for health care services. Simple issues such as eating and drinking sensibly, exercising, and not smoking have been shown to be beneficial to health maintenance. Use emergency facilities only for a true emergency; using emergency facilities for standard care is more expensive and less efficient. Create a safe environment at home to avoid accidents and injuries. Finally, follow your physician's advice; if you don't, you are more likely to require future care, which can be costly and time-consuming.

The choices of a doctor, hospital, and insurance plan have become closely interdependent. Increasingly, the choice of insurer dictates the degree of flexibility you have in choosing the facilities and individuals that will provide medical care for you and your family. All too frequently, people concentrate more on the regular cost of the insurance plan than on what the insurance actually covers. A plan that seems affordable on a monthly or weekly basis can actually cost more over the years if it does not cover the services and procedures your family needs. Though no one can foresee what health care needs will develop over time, your particular situation—a growing family, a chronic condition requiring long-term monitoring or treatment—can be the basis of some reasonable predictions of what kinds of coverage will be most important for you.

The key to making a good choice is to know as much as you can about a health care policy, a hospital, or a doctor before you decide. This requires a lot of homework on your part. It means talking to people that have dealt with the insurance company, the hospital, and the doctor; visiting the various sites and making your own judgments; and defining what you and your family's unique needs are and matching them up with each of these entities. Finally, it means being an informed customer, a prepared patient, and a health-centered individual.

About the Author

Dr. Mike Magee is a nationally recognized physician and leader, described by Richard Knox of the Boston Globe as "the most optimistic physician in America." He is a board-certified surgeon and health care manager, trained at the University of North Carolina and at Ohio State University, and is a nationally known consumer health broadcaster and past president of the National Association of Physician Broadcasters.

Dr. Magee is also an accomplished surgeon and is assistant professor of surgery at Tufts University School of Medicine and the University of Pennsylvania Medical School.

As a health care manager, Dr. Magee created the first U.S. physician-directed hospital department to link community services with physician-patient services. He currently serves as senior vice president of Community and Provider Services at Pennsylvania Hospital and as a consultant to the American Medical Association and the American Hospital Association.

QUESTIONS FOR THE DOCTOR

Q: *My family qualifies for Medicaid, but I have never gotten around to filling out the forms. Can I do this when I get into the hospital?*

A: If you qualify for Medicaid, you are doing your family serious harm by not filling out the paperwork. No one will deny you care, but during a hospitalization, costs can mount rapidly, and whatever money you have could be rapidly used up because of hospital expenses. Medicaid can provide a wonderful service to patients, but, like the government or big-business programs, it is cluttered with complicated procedures. If you are having trouble filling out the forms, take advantage of the services of a hospital social worker or a social worker in your community. These people are trained to help you get through the red tape.

Q: *When I go to the hospital, do I have to accept the doctor that is assigned to me?*

A: I am assuming that you do not have a private physician and that when you go to the hospital, the doctor who is assigned to take care of patients without physicians is given to you. Certainly, at that point you can request another doctor if you are not happy, but the way to avoid this problem is to seek out a family physician or general internist to be your doctor, just in case you are hospitalized. Many people think they do not need a doctor because they are healthy; however, illness is unpredictable and you could end up in a hospital when you least expect it.

There are several reasons why you should have your own doctor. Having your own doctor provides a feeling of comfort. It is nice to know that you have established a relationship with someone who is going to be treating you at a time of serious health concerns for you and your family. All of us have health problems that need to be noted when we go to the hospital, and it is better to have a doctor who knows them in advance. For instance, say your blood pressure is normally low. Most people have a blood pressure of 120 over 80, or thereabouts. If your pressure normally is 108 over 60, that is normal for you and is certainly nothing to be concerned about; but if you go to the hospital after experiencing severe headaches and your blood pressure is 142 over 100, the doctor in the emergency room might think that you have a slightly elevated blood pressure. But for you, that is a severe elevation. There is no way for the assigned doctor in the emergency room to know this unless he or she happens to be your physician or can contact your regular physician. In addition, your regular doctor can order routine screening tests in order to avoid problems before they occur. After all, prevention is the key to maintaining good health.

Q: *I am frustrated. My company has made me switch my HMO [health maintenance organization] three times in the past five years, and each time I have had to get a new doctor. Is there anything I can do about this?*

A: Well, you always have the option of private insurance, but in many cases, the cost is so great that it is not worth the expense. Believe it or not, physicians are feeling the same frustration. Patients that we have known for years switch doctors for economic reasons, understandably so; but the bond that is developed over years of treating a person or his or her family is broken, at least in the professional sense. I don't think is a simple solution, but, clearly, one of the greatest strengths in medicine, the doctor-patient relationship, can be severely strained by this aspect of HMOs. A good aspect of the HMO system, however, is the importance that this system places on prevention and early detection of disease. In fact, many studies have shown that early detection saves lives.

There is no simply solution to this problem, but you should mention the difficulty you are having to your physician and to your HMO. You are not alone in your frustration.

Q: *Why don't doctors make house calls any more?*

A: Actually the number of house calls is beginning to increase, largely because people are being discharged from the hospital earlier than they used to be. When house calls were at their peak, in the 1950s, 10 percent of doctors made house calls. A 1991 study showed that about 2 percent of doctors made house calls; this may not sound like a lot, but it is the highest level in years and it is expected to increase. As health care reform strengthens the role of health consumers, you and other patients will likely have a role in defining what type of care is delivered in the home in contrast to what is delivered in the hospital.

9

Heart Health and Disease

Alfred A. Bove, M.D., Ph.D.

The heart is a muscle that is responsible for distributing blood and oxygen to all parts of the body. Any interference with the heart's function jeopardizes the entire body. Disorders of the heart and blood vessels account for most of the deaths from sickness in the United States. These organs do not go bad by themselves. Usually there is an underlying cause, such as high blood pressure, high cholesterol, smoking, or diabetes. Once a blood vessel is damaged, it can narrow. Once it is narrowed, less blood gets around the body, and this can lead to heart attack, stroke, and the death of tissue in the arms and legs. There are other possible problems as well. This chapter, an overview of heart and circulatory system problems, offers readers suggestions for protecting themselves against heart disease.

Risks for Heart Disease

Risk factors for artery disease are controllable, for the most part, so your heart's health is largely in your own hands. If you smoke cigarettes, are overweight, have elevated blood cholesterol, have high blood pressure, use cocaine, or do not exercise, you are likely to have a heart attack. Combining these risky behaviors can rapidly accelerate atherosclerosis and the aging of your arteries; for this reason even people in their twenties are not immune to heart attack. You can greatly reduce your risk of artery damage by eliminating these behaviors. The most important risk

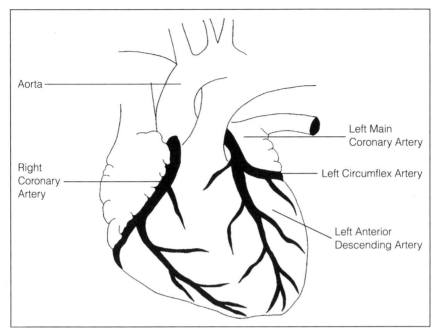

Anatomy of the Coronary Arteries

factor to eliminate is cigarette smoking. Each year some $50 billion in medical bills result from cigarette smoking. Much of that cost is related to treating damaged blood vessels to the heart, brain, and legs, in addition to treating lung cancers that result from smoking.

The levels of blood lipids, fats that are carried in the blood, are also an important risk factor. Cholesterol is a good indicator of the problem. A blood cholesterol level around 200 units is considered safe; levels above 250 increase the risk of heart attack considerably. High blood pressure is another significant risk. Blood pressure should be regularly monitored. Unacceptably high blood pressure can be controlled with medication.

Cocaine use is now known to have a variety of adverse health effects, including damage to arteries. Avoiding cocaine use is an important means of protecting your arteries from damage. Though family history affects your risk of heart disease, it by no means condemns you to repeat the risky behaviors of a preceding generation. Family tendencies to high cholesterol, diabetes, obesity, cigarette smoking, and lack of exercise can be negated by taking charge of your health and by asserting your independence from dangerous practices.

High Blood Pressure (Hypertension)

Blood pressure, the force of blood present in the arteries of the body, is generated by the heart and is the driving force that delivers blood to the tissues and organs of the body. Because the heart is a cyclic pump that thrusts blood into the circulatory system about seventy times per minute, the blood pressure has a periodic pulse that can be felt if a finger is placed over an artery close to the skin. The pulse count is the rate of the heart beat, determined by the pulses within the arterial system. The blood pressure is usually given as two numbers, one "over" the other. The upper number, the *systolic* blood pressure, is the pressure generated by the heart; the lower number, the *diastolic* pressure, is the pressure inside the arteries during the resting phase of the heart beat. (Blood pressure cannot be measured by touching the artery. A blood pressure gauge is necessary.) More than twelve million Americans are affected by high blood pressure. Most specialists consider high blood pressure to be a diastolic (bottom number) that is greater than 85 on three separate occasions in successive visits to the doctor. There is also concern when the systolic (top number) is greater than 160.

Although high blood pressure can have many serious consequences, it can remain undetected for many years if people do not have regular medical examinations. Even when it is detected early, many people do not take their prescribed medication. Because high blood pressure often does not have any immediate symptoms and because blood pressure medications can have annoying side effects (such as depression, fatigue, uncontrolled coughing, or impotence), people think they can do without the medication. But make no mistake, uncontrolled blood pressure can cause severe damage to the heart and kidneys, as well as to the blood vessels feeding the brain and heart. Damage to these blood vessels increases one's risk for stroke and heart attacks. Damage to blood vessels can also affect the arteries that lead to the arms and legs by narrowing the blood vessels and reducing the blood supply to the limbs. In the most severe cases, tissue dies and amputation might be necessary. Another long-term effect of hypertension is reduced exercise tolerance, from the excess load on the heart during ordinary levels of exercise. For some people, even customary activities become too taxing.

Lowering high blood pressure to normal levels is an important health measure to reduce the risk of heart attack, stroke, and kidney damage.

Therefore, it is important to monitor the blood pressure and then to accept the prescribed treatments. In many instances, mild hypertension can be treated by reducing salt intake, body weight, alcohol intake, and cigarette smoking, and by exercising regularly.

These measures can successfully lower high blood pressure, with no further treatment and with diligent health maintenance. However, if blood pressure is severely elevated or if these initial efforts are unsuccessful, treatment must include medication. A variety of blood pressure medications are available. Often, using combinations of them proves more successful than using a single medication alone. Because people differ so much, combinations of medications that are suitable for controlling blood pressure in one person might not be suitable for another, and because blood pressure medications can cause different types of unwanted reactions in some individuals, the physician might have to try different combinations and doses to tailor treatment for each individual.

Cigarette Smoking

I cannot emphasize enough the harmful effects of cigarette smoking. Among the numerous diseases produced by cigarette smoking are atherosclerotic injury to blood vessels, cancer of the lungs and mouth, damage to the lung structure (such as emphysema) and the arteries, which results in heart attacks and strokes. These complications of cigarette smoking are the results of many years of abuse. The increase in blood pressure and heart rate known to be caused by smoking is probably caused by inhaling nicotine or similar products, which directly affect the nerves responsible for regulating the heart and blood vessels. Cigarette smoke also irritates the airways, causing spasm of the upper airways and excess mucus secretion.

Cigarette smoking has a double punch because it not only causes immediate and longer term damage to the lung but also affects blood vessels; especially important are the blood vessels of the heart. Recent research has demonstrated that cigarette smoking causes spasm of the blood vessels of the heart and reduction of blood flow to the heart muscle. This series of events results in oxygen starvation of the heart muscle. This, in itself, can lead to further damage or injury to the heart muscle. The long-term effects of cigarette smoking are now known to contribute to the process of atherosclerosis. Long-term cigarette smokers (fifteen to twenty years) have a very high incidence of coronary artery disease and, consequently, heart attack, sudden death, or chest pain related to heart abnormalities. These events occur because cigarettes seem to increase the speed of damage to blood vessels. Scientists do not know exactly how cigarettes interact with the blood vessels to cause coronary artery disease, but the statistics from many epidemiologic studies clearly show that cigarette smoking is related to blood vessel disease.

Detection and Prevention

The narrowing of an artery can go undetected for a long period of time because it does not yet interfere with blood flow and oxygen delivery to the heart. Only when the artery is 70 percent to 80 percent narrowed will there be evidence of inadequate oxygenation of the heart at rest.

Coronary Artery Disease

Whether it is called *atherosclerosis* or *hardening of the arteries,* coronary disease inevitably causes some individuals to experience a heart attack or require bypass surgery or balloon angioplasty. If they understand the disease and its risk factors, individuals can take measures to avoid the likelihood of coronary disease as they get older.

The process that causes narrowing and, ultimately, the clogging (occlusion) of arteries to the heart, brain, and other organs still is not well understood. Scientists have identified certain risk factors that increase the likelihood of disease, but they do not know precisely how these factors are related to artery damage. Somehow they result in an artery injury, which ultimately leads to a *plaque,* a buildup of debris, in the artery wall. The plaque grows slowly until it damages the inner lining of the artery and encroaches on the opening of the blood vessel enough to impede the flow of blood. The sudden blockage with a clot stops the blood flow and causes the heart muscle supplied by the blocked artery to die. (Remember, the heart muscle needs a blood supply, as does any other organ.) This is the essence of a heart attack. Each year over one million people have a heart attack, and over half of them die suddenly.

Most of the sudden deaths that occur in sports and recreation are because of a heart attack. Occasionally, we hear about a person over age forty dying suddenly while exercising. The most common reason is a heart attack, with an accompanying fatal rhythm called *ventricular fibrillation.* If a person with undetected heart disease jogs, plays tennis, swims, or engages in a strenuous sport, he or she is at risk for sudden cardiac death. The common factor is exertion, which causes the heart to work beyond its capacity to obtain oxygen. The lack of oxygen (called *ischemia*) causes the heart to malfunction and a fatal heart attack to occur.

To test for narrowing before the onset of symptoms, doctors usually stress the patient's heart by having him or her exercise on a bicycle or treadmill. By stressing the heart, physicians can detect loss of blood flow reserve. Injecting a small amount of isotope into a vein allows us to measure the actual blood flow distribution to the heart muscle. When an artery is partially narrowed, we find a lack of flow to the affected area. Physicians also monitor the electrocardiogram (ECG) and blood pressure during the stress test. Abnormalities in the ECG indicate an inadequate flow of blood to the heart. Early in the atherosclerotic process, no symptoms are present in the physical exam, and the ECG may be perfectly normal; but these findings are no guarantee that there is no coronary disease. If you are physically active and over age forty, you should have a periodic stress test to be sure that it is safe for you to exercise.

Prevention is still the most important strategy for long-term health; it involves a commitment to good health and avoidance of obvious harmful habits. Your family history is a clue that you may be at risk for coronary heart disease. If a member of your immediate family (parent, brother, or sister) had a heart attack before age fifty-five, you are likely to be at increased risk. Everyone should have his or her blood lipids (cholesterol, triglycerides, HDL, LDL) measured. If they are abnormal, get advice from your doctor on getting the levels back to normal. Cholesterol should be less than 200 and triglycerides less than 120.

If your blood lipids are not in these ranges, you should lose weight, reduce the saturated fat and alcohol in your diet, and exercise in order to improve these measurements. If these measures do not sufficiently improve blood lipid readings, a physician can prescribe one of several medications that can supplement your efforts to reduce your blood lipids to acceptable levels.

Heart Failure

Another common form of heart disease is heart failure. The problem occurs when the pumping function of the heart is reduced by disease and not enough blood is pumped through the body to sustain its vital functions. Damage to the heart can occur from a wide variety of sources, including heart attacks, viral infections, and too much alcohol consumption. Signs of heart failure are shortness of breath with exercise, lung congestion, swelling of the feet and ankles, and awakening at night with severe breathing difficulties. As heart failure progresses, the kidneys are affected and begin to malfunction. Sometimes the liver is congested enough to malfunction. Finally, when the heart cannot pump enough blood to the brain, mental function is affected.

Usually, the heart damage that reduces the pump function is irreversible. In a small portion of patients, the heart recovers and pump function returns to normal or near normal. The more common situation is the permanent impairment of heart function. Treatment is often designed to reduce the load on the heart (lowering blood pressure, for example), since the damaged heart muscle is usually not able to improve its function greatly.

New medications that lower blood pressure have allowed many patients with heart failure to live near-normal lives; however, there is little therapy available that can improve the long-term outlook for patients with severe heart damage (the major exception is a heart transplant). For these people, treatment usually consists of prescribing several medications that improve the pumping function as much as possible, help remove excess fluid from the body, and lower the load by lowering the blood pressure that the heart must pump against. When medications fail and the heart is severely damaged, patients are considered for *heart transplant*. In this procedure, the heart from a person who has died from an illness or injury that does not affect the heart replaces a patient's severely diseased heart. A person with a transplanted heart can lead a near-normal life with good exercise tolerance and no limitations produced by the failing heart. They must take medications to prevent immune rejection of the donor heart, and they are often prone to hypertension and high cholesterol, which can contribute to the clogging of arteries in the new hearts. In spite of the complex care needed after heart transplant, many recipients are leading productive lives with the heart of another person beating inside their chests.

Mitral Valve Prolapse

As one of the valves that controls blood flow inside the heart, the *mitral valve* can be implicated in several types of heart abnormalities and, in rare situations, in heart disease. Located between the main pumping chamber of the heart, the left ventricle, and the priming pump, the left atrium, the mitral valve acts as a gate, allowing blood to flow in one direction but closing when blood attempts to flow in the reverse direction. The mitral valve itself is made of thin, tough tissue and is supported by fine, sinewy cords that attach to the heart muscle that makes up the walls of the left ventricle. The valve snaps shut every time the heart beats, producing one of the characteristic sounds of the heart.

Several diseases can affect the mitral valve. In the past, *rheumatic fever* was known to damage the valve and produce a lifelong disability because of the narrowing or leakage of the valve. Because of antibiotics, this disease is now rare in the United States, but other infections can damage the valve and cause it to leak. Occasionally, severe chest trauma (as might occur in an automobile accident, for instance) can tear the valve when blood suddenly surges against it. The mitral valve may also function abnormally after a heart attack injures the heart muscle that holds the cords supporting the valve. Abnormal narrowing or leakage of the mitral valve always produces a murmur, which can be heard with a stethoscope.

Mitral valves also vary in size, and in some people that valve seems to be a bit too big for the heart it is in. When this occurs, there is some redundancy of the valve tissue and the valve can balloon into the left

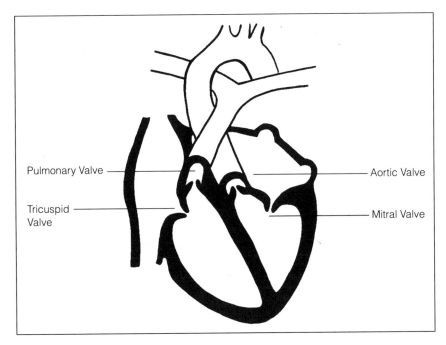

The Valves of the Heart

atrium during the heart beat when the pressure in the ventricle is high. It is this ballooning backward of the mitral valve, which has redundant leaflet tissue, that is called *mitral valve prolapse* (MVP). When this happens, the heart makes a clicking sound, which can be heard with a stethoscope. Today, ultrasound imaging of the heart (echocardiography) has advanced to the point where a clear picture of the mitral valve leaflets can be observed continuously as the heart beats, using a small sound probe that is placed on the front of the chest.

Once the mitral valve could be seen, physicians realized the MVP was very common in healthy people. Current data indicate that 7 percent to 10 percent of all people have mitral valve prolapse. The great majority of them have no evidence of heart disease.

Although MVP by itself cannot be called a disease, a number of heart abnormalities are sometimes associated with this condition and cause physicians to be vigilant for the appearance of other problems. Among the heart problems associated with MVP are palpitations, rapid heart beat, chest pains, and heart murmur. These disorders, it should be stressed, are found in a small minority of people with MVP.

Of these related disorders, the sensation of *palpitations* is the more common. Palpitations are the result of extra heartbeats that occur out of rhythm with the normal heartbeat. When they become bothersome, treatment can be provided with a variety of medications. Occasionally, a person with MVP may have a *rapid heart beat* (tachycardia), although many people without MVP also have this problem; treatment with medication is usually successful in either case. *Chest pain* occurs in some people with MVP. The cause of the pain is not known, but it is not related to angina from a blockage of an artery to the heart. There have been a few reports of more serious heart rhythm abnormalities due to MVP, but these are extremely rare.

About half of those with MVP have a minuscule leak of the mitral valve, which has no effect on the heart. Rarely, the leak becomes significant and the mitral valve must be repaired or replaced. Physicians usually advise people with a leaking valve to take antibiotics when having dental work done, to eliminate the risk of infection of the valve. Bacteria from the mouth could be a possible cause of infection. There is no need to follow this rule if there is no leak of the valve. Similar advice is given to patients with a leak of other valves.

About the Author

Dr. Alfred A. Bove has served as the Bernheimer Professor of Medicine and chief of the section of cardiology at Temple University School of Medicine in Philadelphia since 1986. Prior to this appointment, Dr. Bove was a professor of medicine at the Mayo Medical Clinic from 1981 to 1986, where he also served as a research associate at the graduate school of medicine in 1970–1971.

Dr. Bove earned a bachelor's degree in electrical engineering from Drexel University (1962), and a medical degree (1966) and Ph.D. (1970) from Temple University School of Medicine, where he was also a summer research fellow and research assistant from 1960 to 1966. He completed an internship, residency, and fellowship at Temple University Hospital from 1966 to 1970.

Dr. Bove is a fellow of the American College of Physicians and the American College of Cardiology. He is an established investigator and research committee member of the American Heart Association, where he attained fellow status in the association's councils on clinical cardiology and circulation.

QUESTIONS FOR THE DOCTOR

Q: *I was watching a football game Sunday afternoon, and during the third quarter I experienced a pressure in my chest. I really thought I was having a heart attack, but the pressure lasted only for about a minute and then disappeared. Is this something I should worry about?*

A: Any time you have chest pain, it is something you should be concerned about, at least to the point of calling your physician. There are a number of things that could have happened to you. The most disturbing is that you may have suffered from a bout of angina. In its simplest terms, *angina* is chest tightness and pain because of a decreased supply of oxygen to the heart. Basically, the heart is screaming out for more oxygen and you feel pain. The vessels that supply the heart, the coronary arteries, can become blocked by a wide variety of causes. If, in fact, there was a blockage for one of these reasons and not enough oxygen-carrying blood got to your heart, you would feel this pain.

A heart attack is nothing more than a similar situation, but it is a prolonged episode in which the blood vessels that go to the heart do not open quickly enough, and not enough oxygen-rich blood can get through. When you have a heart attack, heart muscle actually dies and forms a scar. That's why, when you experience chest pain, it is very important to call your doctor or go to an emergency room. Whatever you do, you want to try to minimize as much scar damage as possible.

But you may not have had a heart problem at all. Perhaps you were eating or drinking too much, and you experienced reflux. Extra acid builds up in the stomach and actually pushes out into the esophagus, the tube that connects the mouth to the stomach. The esophagus does not have a very strong lining, and acid can cause aggravation and pain.

There are a host of other problems that can cause chest pain, such as, stress, viral infections, arthritis, and even damage to one of the intercostal muscles that are found between each rib. Once again, if you experience chest pain, call your doctor.

Q: *What is the present thinking about taking aspirin to avoid heart disease?*

A: According to current information, the medical profession favors the administration of one-half aspirin daily to men over age thirty-five. In large population studies, the incidence of heart attacks was reduced by this treatment. Unfortunately, we do not have as many studies to support this treatment in women, although many physicians think it is reasonable to include them in this group. However, before you begin taking aspirin on a regular basis, you should consult your doctor, because aspirin is not a harmless medication. In fact, there is a running joke in the medical profession that if aspirin had to be approved by the FDA today, it might never get approval for use as a drug because of all of its side effects. For instance, if you have any problems with bleeding, aspirin can make the problem worse because of its effect on the platelets. Once again, you and your doctor should decide whether you should take aspirin daily, even though the drug does not require a prescription.

Q: *My doctor wants to put me on a beta-blocker. What is he talking about?*

A: Beta-blockers interfere with specific actions of adrenaline on beta one and beta two receptors, which are found in the blood vessels and heart muscle cells. These beta receptors help to determine heart rate, blood pressure, and just how strongly the heart contracts. Beta-blockers can help lower blood pressure and may even decrease angina episodes. There are a number of beta-blockers on the market, and the class of drugs is quite popular. There are many side effects to beta-blockers, however, including fatigue and impotence; that is why you should consult your doctor. He or she will want to monitor your condition not only when you first get the medication but also in the months following the start of the drug.

Q: *My doctor put me on a calcium channel blocker. He says it is the best drug for me. What do you think about these drugs as a group?*

A: Your doctor knows you best and certainly knows what drug is best for you. I can only speak for the public in general, since I have never examined you. I can tell you this, however, since the calcium channel blockers have come on the market, physicians have had an opportunity to widen broadly their scope of treatment of heart disease and hypertension. Calcium plays a vital role in the pumping of the heart. These medications have one common property: They block the entry of calcium into the smooth muscle of blood vessels and certain heart cells. Calcium channel blockers can help treat people with angina and blood pressure problems, but there are some disadvantages to their use. Certain members of this drug group can cause constipation, palpitations, and light-headedness, but pharmaceutical companies are working on newer forms to decrease these problems.

Q: *I have been diagnosed with heart block. Can this be life-threatening?*

A: If your doctor diagnosed you with this problem and is comfortable with not adding any new medications or devices, your heart block is probably one of the easier ones to deal with. *Heart block* is a delay of the transmission of impulses between the chambers of your heart. The heart is like a huge electrical system, with conduction forces going back and forth over and over again. When the path of this "electrical" current between the atrium and the ventricle is disturbed, you may experience a heart block. There are specific areas along the heart where this can occur. The problem is usually found in the atrioventicular conduction system (the electrical system of the heart). Doctors now have sophisticated electrophysiologic testing methods that can help to evaluate the nature of heart block.

Q: *What is tachycardia?*

A: Tachycardia is a heart rate greater than one hundred beats per minute. The normal heart rate is between sixty and one hundred beats per minute. To take your own pulse, place the index finger of your right hand at the inside of your left wrist on the thumb side, lightly push around that area until you locate a pulse. Count the number of times your pulse beats in one minute. That is your heart rate. If it is over one hundred, you should consult your doctor. Remember, however, that your heart rate may go over one hundred when you are excited or when you are exercising. It will soon return to its normal rate. You should be concerned if your heart rate is constantly elevated, even when you are resting.

Q: *I have used drugs for several years, and my doctor says I have done damage to my heart. How could abusing drugs have affected my heart?*

A: You may have suffered from a bout of *infective endocarditis,* an infection of the cardiac valves or of the endocardium, which lines the heart. The valves that push blood from one side of the heart to the other and push blood from the heart to the rest of the body are often involved because these valves are vulnerable to outside infections. If your damage is great enough, you may need an artificial heart valve. If you have used cocaine, you may have directly damaged the heart muscle or the blood vessels of the heart.

Q: *I've already had one heart attack. What is the best way to avoid a second heart attack?*

A: Research points to some things that can help you prevent another heart attack. If you are a smoker, stop. Have your doctor measure your triglycerides and cholesterol levels on a regular basis. You should also watch your weight and have your blood sugar levels monitored. If you find that you are under too much stress, just don't allow it—your life is too important. You need to take strides to decrease stress.

   If your doctor says that it is all right for you to do so, I suggest that you exercise. Exercise is wonderful; it can be your best friend in a battle like this. Certain drugs, such as beta-blockers and aspirin, can also help you. Once again, check with your doctor.

Q: *My doctor says I need a stress test. What is a stress test, and will it be difficult for me?*

A: Exercise stress testing is a wonderful diagnostic tool that doctors can use to see how well a patient's heart responds to stress. You can have your stress test done on either a bicycle or a treadmill. While you are exercising, your blood pressure is consistently monitored, and your heart's electrical pattern is viewed on a monitor to detect any lack of oxygen to the heart. You will be asked to work yourself to the point of fatigue, but remember, there are health professionals there to watch you and take care of you if there are any problems. There are certain people who should have stress tests; this includes people who have chest pain and people who have a family history of heart attacks and are considered to be at risk. Also, people who have irregular heart beats or want to begin an exercise program are candidates for a stress test as well.

Q: My doctor used a holter monitor to evaluate a fainting episode. What does this monitor do?

A: A *holter monitor* is used to get a reading of your heart beat over a prolonged period of time, usually twenty-four hours. Doctors use the monitor to see if and when irregular heart beats or heart blocks occur. The test is not always successful at detecting problems because people can often go a long period of time without having irregular heart beats or heart blocks. The doctor is trying to catch the problem while it is occurring, and this is much like catching a thief in the act of a crime.

Q: Are birth control pills dangerous for my heart?

A: Birth control pills are much safer than they used to be, but there are still problems. Women who take them for a prolonged period should check with their doctor on a regular basis. If you have a history of blood clots, if you are a smoker, or if you are over age thirty-five, you definitely should check with your doctor to have your birth control pills and continued use evaluated.

Q: Can diabetes make my heart disease worse?

A: There is no doubt that heart disease can be worsened by diabetes because both diseases can contribute to the clogging in blood vessels, including the blood vessels that lead to the heart. If you control your blood sugar, however, you can decrease, or maybe even eliminate, many of these effects. Make certain that you do all you can to monitor your blood sugar levels on a regular basis.

Q: Do you have any tips to keep a healthy heart?

A: My tips are much the same as those of the American Heart Association. They include the suggestions to exercise regularly, eat a diet in which 30 percent or less of calories come from fat, and do not smoke. These three things go hand in hand in improving the life span of your heart and, obviously, your own life span. Regular exercise conditions the muscles of the body so that they demand less of the heart during subsequent exercise. This benefits both the healthy and the sick heart and improves the ability to exercise safely.

10

Nutrition and Disease Prevention

Cheryl Clifford Marco, R.D.

Your eating habits have a great deal to do with the way you look and feel. Healthy eating habits will help decrease your risk of developing coronary artery disease, high blood pressure, stroke, diabetes, pulmonary disease, osteoporosis, and various types of cancer. If you have healthy eating habits, you will feel better every day and you will optimize your performance of daily activities. Food has six nutritional components: carbohydrates, proteins, fats, water, vitamins, and minerals. Of these six, only the first three provide calories. (A *calorie* is the unit used to measure the energy value of the food we eat.)

Calories

People tend to be very concerned about the number of calories consumed every day. The total number of calories you eat is important, but the type of food from which you derive these calories is equally important. With the proper food choices, you can obtain more food value for your calories. This is referred to as *caloric density*.

Of the three nutrients that provide calories, carbohydrates and proteins each provide four calories for one gram of food consumed, but fats provide nine calories for one gram. This illustrates that fat is more calorically dense than is either carbohydrate or protein. The same amount of fat provides more than double the calories of these two types of nutrients.

The determination of a person's calorie need is often oversimplified by plugging height, weight, and activity level into a formula. This gives a rough estimate of calorie needs, but there is a great deal of individual variation. An individual's calorie needs are based on his or her height, weight, age, gender, activity level, body composition, genetics, and possibly past dieting history. Some studies have shown that chronic dieting may decrease an individual's calorie requirements. The most effective way to determine your calorie needs is to keep a record of everything you eat for several days and then to calculate the number of calories you are eating each day. Assuming that your weight is stable, this number is your maintenance calorie requirement. A registered dietitian or a calorie book can help you determine this number.

With regard to weight reduction, however, the number of calories you need a day is not very important. If you want to lose weight, you need to decrease slightly what you are eating or increase your activity level. (If you want to gain weight, you need to increase your typical caloric intake somewhat.) There are thirty-five hundred calories in one pound of fat; therefore, to lose one pound of fat you must eat thirty-five hundred fewer calories than you need for maintenance. Obviously, it is not possible to lose or gain a pound of weight a day. Nevertheless, for each thirty-five hundred calorie deficit below your maintenance calorie needs you will lose one pound of fat.

No matter what level of calories you need to eat a day, it is important to decrease your intake of fats and increase your intake of complex carbohydrates. Your body efficiently stores fat calories as body fat and turns carbohydrate calories into usable energy.

Fats and Cholesterol

The typical American diet derives 38 percent to 40 percent of its calories from fat. All major health organizations recommend that fat intake be decreased to 25 percent to 30 percent of total calories. In order to lower your blood cholesterol level, decrease your risk for developing heart disease and certain types of cancer, and lose weight, it is important to decrease your total fat intake.

Researchers have distinguished three different types of dietary fat: saturated, polyunsaturated, and monounsaturated fat. All fats have the same number of calories, but saturated fats have a more detrimental effect on your blood cholesterol level than do unsaturated fats; therefore, monounsaturated and polyunsaturated fats are preferable.

Saturated Fat

Saturated fats are usually hard at room temperature. Saturated vegetable fats are found in solid, or hydrogenated, shortenings, in coconut oil, palm oil, palm kern oil, and in cocoa butter. (*Hydrogenated* refers to the process of changing an oil from its natural liquid state to a solid state. A product may be partially hydrogenated or completely hydrogenated. For example, margarine is made from hydrogenated vegetable oil that could be completely or partially hydrogenated.) Saturated fats are also found in meat.

Saturated fat increases the amount of cholesterol in circulation, therefore contributing to plaque formation. For this reason, margarines made from completely hydrogenated vegetable oils should be avoided. Read the ingredient label when purchasing margarine to be sure that the first words in the list of ingredients are "liquid vegetable oil," as opposed to "partially hydrogenated vegetable oil."

Saturated fats make up 15 percent to 20 percent of the calories in the American diet but should make up no more than about 10 percent of the calories.

Polyunsaturated Fat

Polyunsaturated fats are found in liquid oils of vegetable origin, such as corn, cottonseed, safflower, sesame seed, soybean, and sunflower oils. There is no evidence that polyunsaturated fats have the same negative effect on blood cholesterol that saturated fats have, but they still contribute a lot of calories. Polyunsaturated fats should make up no more than 10 percent of the calories in the diet.

Monounsaturated Fat

Oils rich in monounsaturated fats include olive oil, canola oil (rapeseed oil), peanut oil, and avocado oil. Recent evidence suggests that olive oil and canola oil may have a beneficial, lowering effect on blood cholesterol levels. (People from Mediterranean regions consume a diet that is relatively high in fat, but a larger percentage of that fat is in the form of olive oil. These populations have a lower incidence of heart disease.) Peanut oil and avocado oil are high in monounsaturated fat but have more saturated fat than does olive oil or canola oil; therefore they have a neutral effect on blood cholesterol levels. It is recommended that

Americans consume 10 percent of their calories from monounsaturated fats.

Cholesterol

Cholesterol is a waxy material manufactured by the body and also present in our diet in foods of animal origin. There is some evidence that the body handles the cholesterol it manufactures differently from the way it handles the cholesterol it consumes. High cholesterol foods include whole milk products such as cream, butter, and whole milk cheeses; egg yolks; organ meats; some cuts of red meat; and shrimp. Cholesterol can be deposited on the artery walls, contributing to atherosclerosis, a process that occurs over a period of time whereby the blood vessels become coated with fatty deposits.

Finding and Limiting Fat

Some of the fat in food is very obvious. It is easily identified in poultry skin, or as the layer of fat that surrounds a steak. The fat in many other foods is less evident. For example, in the fruit and vegetable category, olives and coconuts are high in fat. To reduce and control fat intake, it is important to recognize the most significant sources of fat in your diet. No food should be completely avoided. Instead, reduce your intake of high-fat foods and eat more low-fat foods.

Happily, there has never been a better time to attempt to decrease the amount of fat in your diet. Food manufacturers have responded to the public demand for healthier food by providing a wide variety of low-fat and fat-free products.

Fats in Protein Foods

The major animal and nonanimal sources of protein in the diet are poultry, fish, meat, eggs, cheese, and nuts. There is a wide range of fat content in protein foods; for example, skinless poultry and fish are leaner choices than prime rib or sausage. It is important to choose leaner sources of protein foods more often and to limit your protein intake in general. Americans eat more protein than is necessary, and excess protein is stored as fat.

The following tips will help you limit your fat intake from protein foods:

- Eat no more than six cooked ounces of animal protein foods a day, and include in the six ounces your intake of cheese and eggs. One egg is equivalent to one ounce of protein.

- Before cooking poultry, remove the skin and the layer of fat that lies below it. To keep poultry moist, baste it with broth, wine, frozen juice concentrate, barbecue sauce, mustard, yogurt, or any other low-fat liquid.

- The white meat of poultry contains less fat than the dark meat.

- Smaller chickens (broilers and fryers) are leaner than roasters, which are leaner than hens and capons. Turkey and cornish hens are lean.

- Ground turkey is not always low in fat content because the skin and the dark meat are often included. Have your turkey ground to order from white turkey meat, or purchase turkey labeled "ground turkey breast meat."

- Prepare fish or poultry by poaching in a liquid such as wine, fat-free broth, or vegetable juice seasoned with herbs and spices.

- Buy tuna fish packed in water instead of oil.

- Even though shellfish is high in cholesterol, it is low in saturated fat content, so it does not have as detrimental an effect on blood cholesterol levels as was once thought. But remember to limit total animal protein intake to six ounces a day.

- Trim all visible fat from meat before cooking.

- The Select grade of meat is leaner than the Choice or Prime grades. The leanest cuts of beef are the Select cuts of flank steak, round steak, top round, bottom round, and eye of the round.

- The leanest type of ground beef that you can purchase is Select cuts of round that you have had ground to order. Beware of predetermined fat percentages, since they refer to the fat content by the weight of the product rather than by the percentage of calories from fat. The following describes the percentage of calories that are derived from fat in different grades of ground beef:

73% lean	79% calories from fat
80% lean	71% calories from fat
85% lean	64% calories from fat
90% lean	53% calories from fat
95% lean	34% calories from fat

- Pork is not always high in fat and may be eaten in moderation. The leanest cuts of pork are Canadian bacon, center-cut ham, and pork tenderloin.

- All cuts of veal may be eaten in moderation, with the exception of the veal breast, which is high in fat.

- Brown meats on a rack under a broiler. This allows the fat to drip off.

- When you brown meat on the stove, start with a cold pan and allow the meat to brown gradually. Pour off the fat as it accumulates. If liquid is required, use wine or fat-free broth or another low-fat liquid.

- Keep the amount of processed luncheon meats such as bologna, hot dogs, salami, or sausage in your diet to a minimum. Choose turkey breast, chicken, lean boiled ham, or lean roast beef instead. Luncheon meats and hot dogs made with poultry products are not necessarily low in fat, so read the label carefully.

- Limit the number of egg yolks you eat to fewer than five a week, including those used in recipes. Egg whites are fat and cholesterol free, so you do not need to limit your consumption of them. Two egg whites can be substituted for one whole egg in many recipes. Frozen egg substitutes may also be used, but be sure to choose a brand with no added oil.

- Organ meats are high in cholesterol, so they should be eaten rarely.

- Use tofu and dried beans more often as meat substitutes.

- Peanut butter and nuts are high in fat, so moderate your intake of these foods. When you do eat peanut butter, choose one of the brands that are natural. Natural peanut butter does not have additional fat added, used to prevent peanut butter from separating. The oil separates out in natural peanut butter, so you will need to stir it before each use. You could decrease the fat content of peanut butter even more by pouring off some of the oil on top, but do not pour all of it off because you will not be able to spread the peanut butter.

Fats in Dairy Products

Like protein foods, there is a range of dairy foods, labeled high fat, low fat, and even nonfat. It is important to include dairy products in your diet because they are the best source of dietary calcium, but you should choose low-fat items. There is much confusion about the use of low-fat dairy products. Two percent low-fat milk is lower in fat than is whole milk, but it is still too high in fat to fall within the recommended guideline of deriving less than 30 percent of calories from fat. The term "2 percent" refers to the amount of fat by weight, not by percentage of calories. Therefore, to fall within the recommended guideline for amount of fat consumed, either 1 percent milk or skim milk should be used. The following tips will help you to limit your fat intake from dairy products.

- Gradually switch from whole milk to 2 percent low-fat milk ot 1 percent low-fat milk to skim milk.

- Use cheese sparingly. Low-fat cheese or low-fat cottage cheese may often be substituted for whole milk cheese. Most regular cheese has nine or more grams of fat per ounce; try to choose a cheese with five or less grams of fat per ounce. Cheese should be included as part of your six-ounce daily total of animal protein.

- Cream soups and cream sauces are high in fat. Substitute skim milk for whole milk in recipes and use evaporated skimmed milk in place of cream.

- Use plain low-fat yogurt in place of sour cream or use "mock" sour cream, prepared by blending one cup of 1 percent low-fat cottage cheese with one tablespoon each of lemon juice and skim milk. Allow this to sit in your refrigerator for several hours before using. There are also commercial fat-free sour cream alternatives available.

- Use "yogurt cheese" in place of butter or cream cheese as a spread. You can prepare this by draining plain low-fat or nonfat yogurt in a strainer lined with several layers of cheesecloth. Place the strainer in a bowl and refrigerate overnight. The liquid will drain out of the yogurt and you will have a "cheese" left in the strainer.

- Plain low-fat yogurt or mock sour cream can be used as mayonnaise substitutes in recipes calling for mayonnaise; replace half or more of the mayonnaise with yogurt or mock sour cream. You could also try a commercial fat-free mayonnaise-type spread.

- Try sorbet, fruit ice, sherbet, and low-fat or nonfat frozen yogurt in moderate portions instead of ice cream or ice milk. Frozen desserts made from milk or tofu are not necessarily lower in fat, so read the label carefully.

Added Fats

Added fats are those that are added to your food or used for cooking your food. For the most part, they are not thought of as foods that are eaten alone. Added fats include butter, margarine, mayonnaise, shortening, and oil. Remember that butter and margarine have the same amount of fat, but margarine is usually less of a saturated fat than butter is. It is easy to overlook the added fat in many foods because we really do not think of them as part of our food. For example, mayonnaise-based sandwich spreads, such as tuna salad or chicken salad, usually derive the majority of their calories from fat. Many dessert foods, such as cookies, pies, pastries, and most cakes, also contain a lot of added fat. The following tips will help you to limit your intake of added fats:

- Always measure butter, margarine, oil, and mayonnaise very carefully because small amounts add up to a lot of extra fat.

- Sauté your vegetables (onions, garlic, celery, etc.) in tomato juice, vinegar, wine, vermouth, soy sauce, Worcestershire sauce, fat-free broth, or even in water instead of butter, margarine, or oil.

- Use horseradish, low-fat salad dressing, stewed tomatoes, hot sauce, salsa, mustard, vinegar, lemon juice, catsup, or plain low-fat yogurt on baked potatoes and vegetables.

- Jelly, jam, preserves, or fruit butters may be used instead of butter or margarine as a spread on your bread or food. Try to find one of the pure fruit brands with no added sugar or a low-sugar brand.

- Use nonstick pans and nonstick vegetable oil sprays to decrease or eliminate the need for added fat.

- In recipes that require mayonnaise, replace half of the mayonnaise with plain low-fat or nonfat yogurt. Gradually try to increase the proportion of yogurt to mayonnaise.

- When you must use oil, use a heart-healthier oil such as olive or canola oil.

- Plan ahead when preparing soups or stews. Cook them in advance and allow them to cool so that the excess fat can be skimmed off the top.

- Cook rice and other grains in fat-free broth or juice to give added flavor, thereby eliminating the need to add butter at serving time.

- When using canned broth, put it into the refrigerator overnight before opening. The fat will be hardened on top and can be easily removed.

- Increase your use of herbs and spices as seasonings. This will decrease the need for added fat.

Fats in Breads and Starches

Most breads and starches are not a significant source of fat, but there are a few exceptions. Foods such as biscuits, croissants, pastries, doughnuts, most muffins, and sweet rolls are all high-fat foods. Many of the granola-type cereals are also high in fat.

Most packaged rice and macaroni mixes are high in fat when prepared according to the manufacturers' directions. You can modify the way you prepare them and reduce the fat content. For instance, use skim milk and omit the butter or margarine in a macaroni mix. Increase the amount of milk to replace the butter or margarine. In a rice mix, omit the butter or margarine and use broth, bouillon, or even extra water.

Many crackers are high in fat. In fact, ounce for ounce, most crackers have nearly twice the calories and fat of bread. Avoid crackers advertised as "rich" or "buttery." When purchasing crackers, look for nutritional information; look for no more than three grams of fat for every one hundred calories.

Recommended Fat Limits

Remember that the recommended upper limit of fat a day is 30 percent of your total calorie intake. Consult the following chart for the maximum number of grams of fat you should eat at various calorie levels.

CALORIE LEVEL	MAXIMUM GRAMS OF FAT
1,200	40
1,400	47
1,600	53
1,800	60
2,000	67
2,200	73
2,400	80
2,600	87
3,000	100

You can use package labels as guidelines to tell you the total grams of fat, but be sure that your serving size equals the packager's serving size, or adjust your total up or down accordingly. The Food and Drug Administration (FDA) has recently defined terms that are used on food labels. Before the institution of these definitions, food manufacturers were allowed to interpret a claim by their own standards. The following are the FDA definitions, based on a standard serving size:

LABEL CLAIM	DEFINITION
Calorie Free	Less than 5 calories
Low Calorie	40 calories or less
Light *or* Lite	⅓ fewer calories *or* 50 percent less fat; if more than half the calories are from fat, fat content must be reduced by 50 percent or more
Light in Sodium	50 percent less sodium
Fat Free	Less than ½ gram fat
Low Fat	3 grams or less fat
Cholesterol Free	Less than 2 milligrams cholesterol and 2 grams or less saturated fat

Low Cholesterol	20 milligrams or less cholesterol and 2 grams or less saturated fat
Sodium Free	Less than 5 milligrams sodium
Very Low Sodium	35 milligrams or less sodium
Low Sodium	140 milligrams or less sodium
High Fiber	5 grams or more fiber

It is difficult to determine grams of fat because many of the foods you purchase do not have nutrition labels, especially fresh foods. All packaged foods must carry nutrient-content information, including grams of fat; however, many fresh meats, poultry, and fish do not have the fat content listed on the package, but they still contain fat. If you stop at a bakery for a bran muffin, you may be getting one that has a large amount of fat, but it is difficult to know how large. So, use the package information when it is available, but the best approach is to establish a low-fat life-style. From the information above about where fat is found, begin to choose fewer high-fat foods and more low-fat foods. That way you can reduce your fat intake without spending a lot of time poring over books to look up grams of fat. If you need more specifics, consult a registered dietitian who can individualize and personalize your diet.

Protein

Protein is an essential nutrient of life and is the structural component of all living body cells. Body fluids, enzymes, and hormones are also composed of protein. Although protein is absolutely essential to life, we do not need to eat much protein each day. After the body's basic protein needs are met, it burns excess protein as energy or stores it as fat. Unfortunately, using protein foods for energy is very inefficient, so excess protein is most often stored as fat.

Protein is made up of building blocks called amino acids. In order for the body to make protein that we can use, about twenty different amino acids must be present, in optimal proportions. The body can synthesize the majority of these amino acids; however, there are nine amino acids that are considered *essential;* that is, the body cannot assemble them, so they must be obtained from the food that is eaten. Also, there is no significant storage of amino acids, so foods containing protein need to be eaten regularly.

A protein food is considered *complete* if it contains all nine essential amino acids. Animal protein is generally a complete protein. The sources of animal protein have already been mentioned. There are vegetable sources of protein, but they are considered to be *incomplete* proteins, meaning that one or more of the nine essential amino acids is not present. By combining different vegetable sources of protein in appropriate ways, one can make a complete protein. Vegetable sources of protein include grains, nuts, legumes (dried beans and peas), and vegetables.

It is not difficult to combine vegetable proteins to achieve a complete protein. In fact, the natural way of combining foods usually creates a complete protein. The following combinations will provide a complete protein:

- **An animal source of protein plus a vegetable source of protein.** Even a small amount of animal protein will complement the vegetable protein, making a usable complete protein.

- **A vegetable source of protein plus another vegetable source of protein** (for example, grains plus legumes; grains plus vegetables; nuts or seeds plus legumes; vegetables plus legumes; and vegetables plus nuts or seeds). Note that nuts and seeds do not combine with grains to create a complete protein.

- Some examples of appropriate food combinations are **beans and rice; bread and peanut butter** (peanuts are in the legume family and are not considered a nut); **pasta and beans**; and **bean and vegetable soup.**

As you can see, these are very natural combination of foods, in fact, it is rare that an incomplete protein is eaten on its own.

The Recommended Dietary Allowance for protein is .80 grams per kilogram of body weight, or .36 grams per pound of body weight. The following illustrates how much protein is needed at various body weights:

$$120 \text{ pounds} \times .36 = \text{approximately 44 grams of protein}$$
$$150 \text{ pounds} \times .36 = \text{approximately 54 grams of protein}$$
$$180 \text{ pounds} \times .36 = \text{approximately 65 grams of protein}$$

Most people eat two to three times the protein they need each day. The diet's protein content adds up very quickly. This is illustrated in the following chart, which lists the average grams of protein in various categories of food:

meat, poultry, fish, cheese	7 grams for 1 ounce
eggs	7 grams for 1 egg
milk, yogurt	8 grams for 1 cup
bread	2 to 3 grams for 1 slice
cereal	2 to 3 grams for ¾ cup

pasta, rice	2 to 4 grams for ½ cup, cooked
vegetables	2 to 3 grams for ½ cup
dried beans and peas	7 to 8 grams for ½ cup, cooked
peanuts	4 grams for 1 tablespoon
nuts	3 to 5 grams for 1 ounce

Carbohydrate

The American diet has changed drastically over the past several decades. In the early 1900s, about 60 percent of it was composed of carbohydrate. Although the percentage of carbohydrate has decreased, the percentages of fat and protein intake have increased. The typical diet now consists of only 40 percent to 50 percent carbohydrate, much of which comes from our intake of sugar and foods that are high in sugar.

There are two types of carbohydrates, simple and complex. You should increase your intake of complex carbohydrates and decrease your intake of simple carbohydrates. *Simple carbohydrates* include foods that are quickly digested and absorbed by your body, such as sugar, candy, soda, cookies, cake, pie, and other foods that contain large amounts of added sugar. *Complex carbohydrates* are foods that are digested and absorbed more slowly, including bread, pasta, rice, cereals, potatoes, corn, fruits, vegetables, and dried beans and peas. Complex carbohydrates are good for you, and contrary to popular belief, they are not fattening.

In the discussion of calories, it was explained that carbohydrates provide four calories per gram and fats provide nine calories per gram. Therefore, fats are the most fattening nutrient. Remember that fat should make up 30 percent or less of your diet and that protein should make up 12 percent to 15 percent of your total calories; therefore, carbohydrate should make up the remainder, providing a minimum of 55 percent of your total calories.

Why is carbohydrate important? The major function of carbohydrate in your diet is as an energy source. Our bodies function most efficiently when carbohydrates are the main energy source, rather than fats or proteins. Complex carbohydrates should be included with every meal, especially breakfast. Eating plenty of carbohydrates should increase your energy and performance level. Complex carbohydrates are also the best type of food on which to snack between meals.

Another important role of carbohydrate is to provide fiber. *Fiber* is the material that cannot be digested by your body and is therefore excreted. Unrefined grains are higher in fiber than refined grains; that is, brown rice is higher in fiber than white rice, whole wheat bread is higher in fiber than white bread, and whole grain cereals are higher in fiber than refined cereals. Further examples of whole grain foods are whole wheat bread, whole wheat crackers, whole wheat pasta, rye and oatmeal breads, bran cereals, shredded wheat, barley, buckwheat, bulgur wheat, bran cereals, dried beans and peas, popcorn, fresh fruits, and vegetables. The following are some of the benefits of a high-fiber diet:

- It generally takes longer to eat high-fiber foods, thereby decreasing intake.
- Fiber is very filling; it takes up more space in your stomach and digestive tract than do other nutrients and also absorbs water.
- Fiber decreases intestinal transit time because of the addition of bulk and absorption of water. This helps to relieve constipation.
- A high-fiber diet decreases the incidence of hemorrhoids, diverticulosis, irritable bowel syndrome, and possibly cancer of the colon. This benefit is also because of the decreased intestinal transit time.

Your fiber intake should be increased gradually, because one side effect of a high-fiber diet is flatulence. This can generally be avoided with a gradual increase of dietary fiber and plenty of water.

Sugar

Even though this simple carbohydrate has been touted as "public enemy number one," sugar intake has drastically increased over the past several decades and the complex carbohydrate intake has decreased. Sugar is not the most desirable form of carbohydrate to eat, but neither is it the nutritional enemy that many have claimed.

Sugar provides none of the essential nutrients that our bodies require on a daily basis. About 20 percent of our daily intake of calories is from sugar (and another 40 percent is from fat), so a lot of empty calories are being consumed. Sugar can also be the source of a great number of calories. Sugar itself has only sixteen calories a teaspoon, but there can be a lot of sugar hidden away in various foods, causing the calories to add up. A high-sugar intake, therefore, contributes to obesity, which in turn increases the risk of many other diseases.

When foods that have a high concentration of sugar are eaten on an empty stomach, they may cause a condition called *rebound hypoglycemia*.

You may reach for a candy bar as a midafternoon snack when you are starting to drag, only to feel worse about half an hour after eating it. A sugary food such as a candy bar is quickly digested. The sugar enters your bloodstream and insulin is secreted from your pancreas to lower the level of sugar in your blood. When too much sugar is eaten, however, your blood sugar level may go too low, causing you to feel more lethargic. Our bodies are much more efficient at processing complex carbohydrates that are digested more slowly.

Calcium

Until now, this chapter has been concerned with nutrients that provide calories. Calcium is a mineral and is essential to life, but it does not provide calories. Calcium is found in our bones, teeth, and bloodstream. Although the calcium in our bloodstream constitutes only 1 percent of the total calcium in our bodies, it is necessary for blood clotting, transmission of nerve impulses, muscle contraction, heart function, and activation of enzymes. Our bodies' blood calcium levels will remain stable by pulling calcium from the bones, if necessary.

Osteoporosis is a disease characterized by a gradual loss of bone mass and increased susceptibility to fractures. It is found most often in postmenopausal women. Women are at higher risk for osteoporosis than are men because they have less bone mass than men and because they lose bone density earlier in life than do men. Estrogen levels drop drastically at menopause, which causes an acceleration of bone loss. Women also tend to eat less calcium than men throughout their lives because of a concern with fat and calories.

The amount of bone tissue in the human body increases throughout childhood and adolescence, and, for some bones, even into the thirties. Research has indicated that consuming adequate calcium during this time could prevent or delay the onset of osteoporosis. There is also evidence that adequate calcium intake after this time could slow bone loss that has already started.

Calcium Intake

The RDA for calcium is 1,200 milligrams a day for eleven to twenty-four-year-old males and females and for pregnant and lactating women. It is 800 milligrams for children under eleven and adults over twenty-four. The National Institutes of Health and the National Osteoporosis

Foundation recommend that adults consume 1,000 milligrams of calcium daily. Because estrogen conserves calcium, a postmenopausal woman needs up to 1,500 milligrams daily. (See Table 10-1 for some food sources of calcium.)

As you can see, the best sources of calcium are dairy products. The bones of sardines and salmon are also high in calcium, so it is important to eat them occasionally, too. Some green vegetables are a good source of calcium. Spinach, however, also contains a compound called oxalate, which interferes with the absorption of calcium.

Calcium Supplementation

There are several different forms of calcium, including calcium acetate, calcium carbonate, calcium citrate, calcium gluconate, and calcium lactate. Recent studies have shown that all forms are absorbed similarly and that the absorption rates are also similar to the absorption rate of calcium from milk. Some calcium supplements contain so little calcium,

TABLE 10-1
Sources of Calcium

Food	Serving	Calcium (in milligrams)
Milk		
whole	1 cup	288
skim	1 cup	302
Yogurt, plain, low fat	1 cup	450
Ice cream	½ cup	90
Ice milk	½ cup	90
Cheese		
cheddar	1 ounce	204
cottage, 1% low fat	½ cup	69
cream	1 ounce	23
mozzarella, part skim	1 ounce	183
ricotta, part skim	½ cup	337
Swiss	1 ounce	272
Fish		
sardines with bones	3 ounces	372
salmon, pink, with bones	3 ounces	167
Vegetables		
broccoli	1 cup, cooked	120
collard greens	1 cup, cooked	340
kale	1 cup, cooked	200
spinach	1 cup, cooked	168
turnip greens	1 cup, cooked	252

however, that several tablets must be taken in order to meet daily requirements. Calcium carbonate contains the most calcium per tablet.

A calcium supplement may be needed if you are unable to consume enough calcium in your diet. You may want to rely on dietary sources for some of your daily calcium and use a supplement to make up the difference. Check with your physician before taking a calcium supplement because there are some medical conditions that may contraindicate its use.

Sodium

Sodium, a mineral that is essential to life, is found naturally in many foods. Sodium is found in every body cell. It helps in the transmission of nerve impulses and in muscle contraction. Although the terms "salt" and "sodium" are often used interchangeably, they do not have the same meaning. Salt is sodium chloride, which contains about 40 percent sodium and 60 percent chloride. It is the *sodium*, not the salt, that has been implicated in many health issues.

All Americans would benefit from a reduction in sodium intake. The National Academy of Sciences recommends limiting sodium to no more than 2,400 milligrams a day, though the National Heart, Lung, and Blood Institute advises that sodium be restricted to no more than 3,300 milligrams a day. The typical American consumes 4,000 to 6,000 milligrams of sodium a day. The amount of sodium in one teaspoon of salt is 2,000 milligrams.

It is believed that in normal, healthy adults the typical level of sodium intake poses no health problem because the body eliminates what is not needed. However, a high sodium intake is thought to exacerbate a high blood pressure, or hypertension, in some people. It has not been proven that a high sodium intake causes high blood pressure or that a reduced sodium intake can actually prevent high blood pressure. Therefore, if you have high blood pressure, you should cut back on your sodium intake, but there is probably no need to cut back for preventive reasons. Proponents of across-the-board recommendations to reduce sodium intake argue that it is not harmful in any way to do so. Although this is true, there are other dietary changes that are much more important for all people, such as reducing fat intake and increasing fiber intake.

Sodium occurs naturally in many foods that are not considered salty, such as milk and meat. This amount accounts for approximately one-third of the sodium in our diets. Sodium is also found in table salt, which is added either in cooking or at the table. This amount also accounts for approximately one-third of the sodium in our diets. Processed and salt-cured foods account for the last third. This includes luncheon meats, hot dogs, frozen dinners, canned vegetables, canned soups, potato chips, pretzels, condiments (catsup, mustard, relish, salad dressing), and so on. Eating more fresh foods and preparing more meals "from scratch" will help you to decrease your sodium intake from processed foods.

Vitamins and Minerals

The vitamin and mineral supplement industry is a multimillion-dollar business. Americans generally believe that our diets will become balanced if we add vitamin and mineral supplements. Most of the discussion in this chapter has been centered on the importance of good nutrition in the prevention of disease and in the improved performance of daily activities. You have seen the role that carbohydrate, protein, and fat play in overall health and well-being. This information has been obtained by scientists and researchers who looked at the actual food intake of various groups and populations. You should conclude now that you cannot eat an unhealthy diet and then take a vitamin supplement to correct your mistakes.

Given this, it is still important to consider your daily requirements and the need for vitamins and minerals. The U.S. Recommended Dietary Allowances (RDA) are established guidelines for nutrient needs. The RDA is the numerical expression of the quantity of certain nutrients believed to be adequate to meet the known nutritional needs of practically all healthy people. The allowances were determined by the National Research Council of the Food and Nutrition Board. They were first established in 1943 and have been revised nine times since then, most recently in 1989. Each RDA has been established at a higher-than-average requirement, to allow a safety margin.

It can be a dangerous practice to take vitamin and mineral supplements. Certain levels of vitamins may produce a drug or medication effect. An even higher intake level can actually produce a toxic effect. Both fat-soluble and water-soluble vitamins can be potentially toxic. With minerals, a balance is often necessary for optimal absorption. For example, too much of one mineral may impair absorption of another mineral.

Although there can be toxic and harmful side effects with large doses of vitamins and minerals, there is probably no harm in taking a multivitamin and mineral supplement in the proper amount if you are unable to eat a well-balanced diet. When you purchase a supplement, look for one that provides 100 percent or less of the RDA for the various vitamins and minerals. This information should be available on the label; if it is not, do not buy that supplement. The particular brand you purchase is not important; in fact, the generic brands or the store brands are often just as good as and are less expensive then name-brand products. Always check the vitamins' expiration dates and store the bottles in a cool, dry place, out of direct light. It is important to remember that a vitamin supplement is not a cure-all for a high-fat, low-fiber, high-sugar, high-sodium, low-carbohydrate diet.

Diet and Heart Disease

It is well established that eating a low-fat, low-cholesterol, high-fiber diet can modify your risk for developing heart disease. For every 1 percent decrease in your blood cholesterol level, you are decreasing your risk of developing heart disease by 2 percent. Other factors, such as genetics, gender, and age, play a role in your risk for heart disease, but it is important to change the risk factors that you are able to change. The methods and recommendations for decreasing fat given in this chapter should help many people, but if you find you need or want more specific recommendations, you should see a registered dietitian for personalized nutrition counseling.

Diet and Obesity

Obesity is one of the most prevalent health problems in the United States. It is estimated that one out of four adults is obese. Obesity is the result of a combination of genetic and environmental factors. There are many health risks associated with obesity and overweight, including an increased risk for heart disease, hypertension, gallbladder disease, diabetes, breathing problems, and certain types of cancer. In addition, obesity places a functional burden on the body and may exacerbate certain conditions, such as arthritis.

Recent studies also suggest that fat distribution on the body is even more predictive of morbidity and mortality. Persons with upper-body obesity are at greater risk of disease than those with lower-body obesity. Fat distribution can be objectively measured by a waist-to-hip ratio (WHR). Measure your waist circumference at the level of the navel and the hip circumference at the largest point of the buttocks. In women, a WHR of 0.8 or greater is considered high risk. In men, a WHR of 1.0 or greater is considered high risk.

But how much should you weigh? This determination is not as simple as one might suppose. What you weigh in total pounds is much less important than what your weight is composed of — you can be overweight according to a height-weight table, but you may not be "overfat." People who exercise, particularly those who weight-train, may be overweight, but not overfat. Risk for disease is more closely associated with being overfat than with being overweight. Conversely, your weight may be within normal limits, but you may be overfat, which also increases your risk. To determine whether you are overweight or overfat, you need to have your body composition measured. This can often be done by a registered dietitian or by an exercise physiologist. The following rule-of-thumb formula will give you an idea of what your ideal weight is, but because individuals vary so much it should not be regarded as the definitive gauge.

FEMALES: *100 pounds for the first 5 feet of height*
                                    PLUS
                  5 pounds for each inch of height over 5 feet
          Example: 5'4" tall
          100 pounds + (5 pounds × 4 inches) =
          100 pounds + 20 pounds = 120 pounds

MALES: *106 pounds for the first 5 feet of height*
                                    PLUS
                  6 pounds for each inch of height over 5 feet
          Example: 5'11" tall
          106 pounds + (6 pounds × 11 inches) =
          106 pounds + 66 pounds = 172 pounds

Diet and Cancer Prevention

Certain types of cancer have been linked to diet, although definitive conclusions have not yet been made. Certain foods may increase your risk of cancer, but others may play more of a protective role.

Fat

A high-fat diet has been linked to a higher incidence of breast, colon, and prostate cancers. These are the most common cancers in the United States. The total fat content of the diet is more important than a particular type of fat, so again, the prudent advice is to decrease fat intake.

Salt-Cured, Nitrate-Cured, and Smoked Foods

These types of foods seem to have a carcinogenic (the potential to cause cancer to develop) effect in populations that use them regularly and in large amounts, but they are not proven to be a major contributor to cancer. And although there is no recommendation to avoid charcoal grilling, you should avoid charring foods. Partially precook foods that require a long barbecue time and try to avoid the creation of smoke produced by fat dripping on the coals and rising back up to the meat. Use a squirt bottle to dampen the coals if there is a lot of smoke.

Alcohol

Heavy drinkers seem to have incidence of cancers of the mouth and throat, but there is not an established link. People who drink *and smoke* have an even greater risk for developing cancer. (Alcohol is also high in calories; seven calories per gram of alcohol.)

Fiber

A high-fiber diet plays a protective role against the development of colon and breast cancers. All Americans should increase their fiber intake.

Vitamin C

Vitamin C intake is linked to a lower incidence of cancers of the stomach and esophagus. Foods high in vitamin C include citrus fruits and juices, broccoli, cabbage, cantaloupe, red and green peppers, brussels sprouts, turnip greens, cauliflower, kiwis, and strawberries. Everyone should eat at least one serving of a food rich in vitamin C daily.

Beta-Carotene

Beta-carotene has been linked to lower cancer rates and it may reduce the risk for developing lung cancer. The richest sources of beta-carotene are fruits and vegetables that are deep yellow, orange, or dark green.

These include apricots, broccoli, cantaloupe, carrots, kale, mangos, mustard greens, peaches, pumpkins, spinach, sweet potatoes, tomatoes, and winter squash.

Cruciferous Vegetables

These types of vegetables also seem to offer protection against the development of some cancers. They include broccoli, brussels sprouts, cabbage, cauliflower, kale, rutabaga, and turnip. Some studies show that *indole*, a compound contained in these vegetables, may boost the action of liver enzymes that break down certain carcinogens.

Supplementation

It seems as if the easy answer to preventing cancer, and to maintaining health in general, is to take a supplement with all of the anticancer substances in it. Unfortunately, there is no such supplement available. The evidence that vitamin and mineral supplements prevent cancer is still somewhat unclear. In fact, it may turn out that fruits, vegetables, and whole grains in general, rather than selected substances, are what really play the protective role. Again, a multivitamin and mineral supplement in doses that do not exceed the RDA is probably not harmful for most people, but the best protection against cancer remains a well-balanced, varied diet that is low in fat and high in fiber.

About the Author

Cheryl Clifford Marco's career as a registered dietitian has spanned more than a decade. She is currently the manager of the outpatient nutrition service in the Department of Nutrition and Dietetics at Thomas Jefferson University Hospital in Philadelphia, an institution she joined in 1982 as a clinical dietitian.

Throughout her career, Ms. Marco has endeavored to make nutritional information more accessible to the general public. In conjunction with her colleagues, she has instituted and maintains low-fat cooking classes, individual nutrition counseling, a weight-management program, and the "Dining with Heart" program, which involves working with restaurant chefs to help them develop menu items that are lower in fat, sodium, and cholesterol while still maintaining taste appeal.

Along with her clinical expertise, Ms. Marco is affiliated with local and national professional societies, including the American Dietetic Association, the Pennsylvania Dietetic Association, the Philadelphia Dietetic Association, and the Practice Group of Sports and Cardiovascular Nutritionists. She has been a frequent lecturer to both professional and consumer groups on topics ranging from sports nutrition to obesity.

QUESTIONS FOR THE DOCTOR

Q: *About four months ago I stopped smoking with the help of the nicotine patch. I am surprised at how well I have done so far, but my concern is that I have gained about ten pounds since I stopped smoking. I'm not sure which is worse, smoking or gaining weight. Is it normal to gain weight after a smoking cessation program?*

A: Yes, as a matter of fact, many people gain weight when they stop smoking cigarettes; a person can expect to gain five to ten pounds after quitting smoking. One reason for weight gain is that, for a short period of time at least, the basal metabolic rate decreases. Cigarettes contain nicotine, which acts as a stimulant and increases adrenaline. With an increase of adrenaline comes a more rapid heart rate, an increase of energy, and an increased ability to burn calories; thus, lower weight in smokers. Recent studies have shown that, despite the fact that smokers tend to be thinner than they would be if they were nonsmokers, they have elevated levels of cholesterol and higher levels of LDL, or "bad" cholesterol.

A slight increase in weight is well worth the disappearance of toxic substances in your body. There is no doubt that cigarette smoking has been linked to heart disease and cancer. In addition, cigarette smoke, in its passive form, has also been linked to an increased risk of cancer in family members and in those exposed to the smoke. One final point: although statistics show that there is an increase in weight after quitting cigarette smoking, this does not mean that you have to give up trying to quit. Keep up the good work, and don't get discouraged.

Q: *There is a great deal of information about nutrition in adults, but what about children? Should I be concerned about my baby's cholesterol? Also, should I be worried about giving my baby whole milk?*

A: We are beginning to learn the importance of dietary management in children. Our nation's children are the heaviest they have ever been; in addition, they are in the poorest condition. Although an increase in exercise helps burn calories, for a wide variety of reasons our children are not exercising as much as they used to. One of the biggest culprits is time spent in front of the television set. A recent study showed that children actually burn *fewer* calories when they are watching TV than when they are resting. In addition, advertising on television tends to promote high-fat products, such as candy and cakes. The combination of decreased burning of calories and increased intake of food adds to the weight problem.

Doctors as a whole are not concerned about cholesterol levels in the first two years of a child's life unless there is a strong family history of heart disease and severe pathologic elevations of cholesterol. Cholesterol has a major role in building up the cell walls in many organs, including the brain, so your baby's cholesterol level should not be a major concern now.

Recently, a number of scientists recommended that milk not be given to children in the first two years of life, for a wide variety of reasons, including possible milk allergies. This is a decision you should make with your doctor, but the American Academy of Pediatrics and others who deal with this problem on a regular basis recommend adding whole milk to your body's diet only after the first year. During the first year, breast milk or formula is better, to ensure fortification of vitamins and proper caloric intake.

Q: *I have heard that a high-fat diet can lead to cancer. Is this true?*
A: There is reason to believe that a high-fat diet increases your risk of cancer. Studies in rats have shown that those who are fed a low-fat diet have a dramatically lower incidence of colon cancer than those who are fed a high-fat diet. Other studies have shown a link between a high-fat diet and breast cancer, although the results remain controversial. I agree with the author of this chapter that no more than 25 percent to 30 percent of your diet should be fat calories. Nevertheless, fat is part of a normal diet and you should not be afraid of eating it, but, once again, the key is proportion.

Q: *I take a multivitamin. Is this a good idea?*
A: There is no reason not to take a multivitamin because the body will use the added nutritional support if it needs it. If it does not, it will process the unused vitamins and excrete them in the urine. But make sure that you do not take too many vitamins, because you can suffer a severe toxic reaction to megadoses.

Q: *What do you think about fish oil as a dietary supplement?*
A: Several years ago, there was a major report stating that Eskimos, who consume fish oil as part of their diets, had a decreased risk of heart disease. This report was followed by an explosion in the manufacturing of fish oil products to be used as nutritional supplements. There

is some support to the theory that fish oil can help fight heart disease, but many studies have shown that if people consume too much fish oil, they may actually increase their LDL, or "bad" cholesterol. At the present time, not enough research has been done to support the use of fish oil as a supplement.

Q: *Is oat bran as good as people say at fighting cholesterol and heart disease?*

A: Some studies have suggested that people who eat a great deal of oat bran for breakfast have a decreased risk of heart disease. These people may be substituting oat bran for other foods that could be high in cholesterol, such as eggs or bacon. The evidence is not conclusive concerning the benefits of high-fiber foods, such as oat bran. Once again, you should try to maintain a balanced diet; oat bran is a great fiber food, but it is not a cure-all.

Q: *What do you think about aspartame, the product used in Nutra-Sweet?*

A: This product is now found in so many places and in so many foods that it is almost impossible to avoid. Only people who have a disease called *phenylketonuria* and known to be at risk from exposure to aspartame. At the present time, there is no need for you to be concerned.

I have had people tell me that they worry about aspartame because they drink seven or eight diet sodas per day. They should worry less about the effects of aspartame and more about drinking so many sodas. I think it is fair to say that all foods should be consumed in moderation. Your common sense should warn you that if you find yourself drinking excessive amounts of fluids or eating excessive amounts of food, you need to take a careful look at your diet.

Q: *I love filet mignon. My cholesterol is about 200 and I am forty years old. I have heard that filet mignon and other types of meat are bad for my cholesterol. I really miss it. What can I do?*

A: If you are otherwise healthy and are having a normal range of cholesterol for your age, there is no reason why you cannot occasionally enjoy a treat like filet mignon, even though it is high in fat. The same goes for ice cream or chocolate cake, for that matter. But you must remember not to overdo it.

Q: *I am on a heart medication, and one of the side effects is an interaction with specific foods. Is this interaction common for many medications?*

A: In different situations, certain medications may interact with other medications or with food and cause problems. On the whole, doctors often fall short in counseling patients about problems associated with interactions of drugs and foods. For example, physicians may fail to mention that patients can decrease the effectiveness of tetracycline if they combine it with milk. The milk hinders the absorption of the tetracycline, so not enough is absorbed to help fight the infection for while the tetracycline is being used. Many drugs have similar interaction problems associated with their use. If your doctor does not mention food and drug interactions to you, please ask about them.

Q: *Every time I drink coffee, I get heartburn. I'm not a doctor, but it seems to me that this coffee might be causing this problem. Am I right?*
A: There are many causes of heartburn. If you have been having this problem for a prolonged period (about three weeks or more), you should consult your doctor. Often, all it takes to prevent heartburn is to avoid certain foods. Caffeine, alcohol, aspirin, and tobacco can irritate the stomach and cause a buildup of acid. The acid can extend into the esophagus, the tube that goes from the mouth to the stomach. Because the lining of the esophagus is not strong like the lining of the stomach, a small amount of acid can cause a great deal of pain, perceived as heartburn. In addition, small ulcerations can develop in the stomach lining and in the lining of the small intestine, and these, too, can cause pain. Coffee drinking could be the cause of your difficulty. I suggest that you restrict caffeine products, including coffee, tea, and sodas, but, if your problem continues, you should see your doctor and have it evaluated.

Q: *I get hungry right before my menstrual period. Is this normal?*
A: Hormonal variations during a typical menstrual cycle can vary widely. Increased hunger is associated with the onset of menstruation; it is normal to have increased hunger at this time.

Q: *I used to exercise regularly, but since my knee injury, I have had to stop. I have been gaining weight, although I am eating the same amount of food. Do you have any suggestions?*
A: You should begin some sort of aerobic activity that your doctor approves of, since your knee injury is preventing you from exercising. Exercise, especially aerobic exercise, has been shown to be helpful for the heart, even if you only do it three times a week. It helps burn calories, not only during the period of exercise but also throughout the day. It increases your basal metabolic rate and helps you burn

calories more effectively. I am not surprised that you have gained weight. This may continue to be a problem until you begin some form of exercise. Certainly, you can reduce your intake of calories, but be careful not to reduce them too much. Carefully watch the amount of fat in your diet. If you can reduce it, you will be doing what is most effective to help control your weight.

11

Pregnancy and How It Changes a Woman's Body

Richard Henderson, M.D.

Understandably, pregnancy can be a time of considerable excitement and anticipation as well as apprehension and concern about what might happen. Because there is an enormous amount of material on pregnancy available today, the goal of this chapter is to address the common questions about pregnancy. The discussion begins with the important matter of the mother's health before pregnancy; what happens in this time may be crucial to the well-being of the expectant mother and the pregnancy.

Preconception

Once a woman knows she is pregnant, she usually reviews her life-style and personal habits. But the pregnancy may not have been diagnosed until eight, twelve, or even sixteen weeks have passed, and in that time the fetus may have been unknowingly and unintentionally exposed to potentially harmful agents during these critical weeks of development. The best time to make changes in life-style and personal habits, therefore, is before pregnancy begins. If you smoke, drink, or use drugs, stop before you get pregnant. If you are required to take medicine for a particular condition, take time to discuss both your condition and your medication with your health care provider before pregnancy. Even if you are fond of junk foods, you may need nutritional counseling to help you provide the best nourishment during your pregnancy.

166

Conception

Pregnancy begins when one of millions of sperm penetrates the one egg that has been released from the ovary during an ovulatory cycle. When pregnancy occurs, a complex series of hormonal changes begins. One result of these changes is that the regular cycle of ovulation stops and therefore menstrual periods stop for the term of the pregnancy. Other signs of early pregnancy are increased urination, fatigue, and breast tenderness.

The most reliable and accurate way to find out if you are pregnant is to have a blood pregnancy test. This test is so accurate that it can determine pregnancy even before the first period is missed. The home pregnancy tests available today are more accurate and reliable than in the past, but they are not as reliable as a blood test. A positive home test should be confirmed by a blood test. If the home test is negative but you think it might be wrong—perhaps you just "feel" pregnant—you should have a blood test to resolve the question.

Once pregnancy has been confirmed, the question becomes, How far along am I? *Gestational age,* or the age of the fetus, is calculated by adding from the first day of the last menstrual period. On average, about 280 to 294 days, or 40 to 42 weeks, pass between the first day of the last normal menstrual period and delivery of the infant. For most purposes, the understanding that an average pregnancy lasts 280 days or nine calendar months is more convenient because this period is easily divided into three parts, or *trimesters,* with each trimester lasting three calendar months. Thus, to figure the fetus's gestational age, count the number of weeks that have passed since the beginning of your last period.

Gestation

Gestation is the process of "growing a baby." Within the first twelve weeks of gestation, every major organ system is formed. It is very important for pregnant women to avoid exposure to chemicals and other dangerous products during the first trimester because inappropriate exposure may lead to birth defects. A tremendous amount of growth occurs in the embryo in the first twelve weeks. The eyes, lungs, and heart develop by the beginning of the fifth week, and circulation begins with the development of the heart. The embryo continues to develop and grow. A gastrointestinal system has formed, and by the sixth week, the gonads (ovaries or testes) have differentiated (sex is determined at fertilization). From the eighth week until birth, the embryo is referred to as a *fetus.*

By the midpoint of pregnancy (twenty weeks), the fetus is almost six inches long and weighs about eleven ounces. Growth continues at a dramatic rate, and by thirty-six weeks, the average weight is five and one-half pounds and the fetus is about twelve inches long. (Most babies born prematurely at thirty-six weeks survive and do well.) By forty weeks, the average length is more than fourteen inches and the average weight is seven and one-half pounds.

Body Changes

A woman's body experiences considerable changes as pregnancy advances. These changes are so radical that if they occurred outside pregnancy, one might believe that they were caused by a disease process. The changes that a woman's body goes through in pregnancy, however, are very normal and predictable. Some of the major ones involve the uterus, skin, heart, lungs, gastrointestinal tract, musculoskeletal system, and the hematologic (blood) system.

The uterus rapidly increases in size to accommodate the growing fetus, placenta, and amniotic fluid. Before pregnancy, the uterus appears as an almost solid, muscular structure. During pregnancy, it undergoes changes to become a thin-walled, muscular organ, which is capable of providing an ideal environment for the development of the fetus. After delivery, the uterus demonstrates one of its most remarkable abilities: It contracts to slow and then stop the bleeding that occurs from the womb after birth. If this contraction does not occur, the amount of blood lost during delivery can be life-threatening. The uterus then continues to shrink until it is again normal size by six weeks after delivery.

Changes also occur in a pregnant woman's skin. Often noticeable are irregular brownish patches that may appear on the neck and face, called the "mask of pregnancy," or *chloasma.* Many pregnant women also have considerable darkening of the skin along the midline of the abdominal wall. This darkening line is called the *linea nigra.* The same kind of darkening of the skin may also occur over the entire abdomen. The dark color may lighten in time—taking weeks, months, or even years after delivery to do so—but it usually remains somewhat visible. Similarly, stretch marks, which appear on the abdomen, buttocks, and sometimes the thighs, may be red or darker colored during pregnancy, but they usually lighten after delivery. This may also take some time to occur. There is no specific cream or other agent that will lighten the darkened skin or prevent stretch marks.

Many changes occur in both the heart and the lungs of pregnant women that may produce alarming symptoms or feelings that provoke questions. An expectant mother may notice that her heart beats stronger and faster. This is necessary so that the heart is able to supply more blood, nutrients, and oxygen to the fetus growing in the uterus. Many woman report increased awareness of a desire to breathe. Pregnant women must take more frequent and deeper breaths. This feeling of being short of breath is the result of significant physical changes that are usually felt more in the last few months of pregnancy. Because the abdomen is being physically pushed up against the bottom of the lungs, many women experience these kinds of alterations in their normal breathing patterns.

Everything in the abdominal cavity is being pushed upward by the growing uterus. Many change can occur in the digestive, or gastrointestinal, tract, which begins at the mouth and ends at the anus. The major organs in this system include intestines, stomach, liver, gallbladder, and pancreas. In the mouth, the gums may swell and bleed more easily during pregnancy, even during gentle brushing. A local growth, which looks like a tumor and may bleed heavily, may form on the gums. This is typically not a tumor, and it usually goes away after delivery.

Heartburn is also a frequent problem experienced by women during pregnancy. The physical pressure put on the lower part of the stomach, as well as hormones produced during pregnancy, cause the muscles between the opening of the stomach and the esophagus to relax. This allows some of the contents of the stomach, including digestive acids, to be pushed, or refluxed, up into the esophagus. Refluxing may cause an aching feeling deep behind the chest bone (sternum) or a burning, bitter taste in the back of the mouth. Any antacid should provide relief, but pregnant women should not use products containing sodium bicarbonate because they may cause changes in the body's acid balance.

Many pregnant women develop hemorrhoids because of the pressure placed on the rectum from the enlarging uterus. The pressure slows blood in the veins at the level of the uterus and below it. This causes a buildup in blood pressure and an enlargement in those veins. When a vein in the anal area enlarges and bulges or protrudes and forms a clot, it is called a *hemorrhoid*. (When this pooling of blood occurs in the veins of the leg, it results in varicose veins.) Hemorrhoids may also be caused by constipation, another source of discomfort for expectant mothers. Hemorrhoids sometimes bleed; although any type of bleeding is especially disturbing during pregnancy, this type usually presents no danger to the mother or her fetus. Bleeding from hemorrhoids usually stops without treatment, but it should be reported to your doctor. Hemorrhoids may develop and cause discomfort at any time, but this happens especially during pregnancy. Even women who never had hemorrhoids before may develop them during pregnancy. Women who develop hemorrhoids while they are pregnant usually have them during each pregnancy.

Changes in a woman's muscles and bones (musculoskeletal system) often cause some discomfort as her pregnancy advances. One of the most noticeable changes involves posture. As the uterus gets larger and grows to fill the abdominal cavity, the center of gravity in the lower back shifts so that it is over the bones of the pelvis and legs. This shift, in conjunction with a loosening of the ligaments between the bones of the pelvis caused by hormones made during pregnancy, frequently causes discomfort in the lower back and pelvis, especially in the last trimester. The lower part of the spine is pulled farther forward and alterations occur in the bones of the shoulders and the spine in the neck (cervical spine). To compensate for the change of gravity in the abdomen, the shoulders roll or are hunched forward. As more pressure or strain is placed on the large nerves that come from the cervical spine into the arms, during the last few months of pregnancy a woman may experience aching, numbness, or weakness of the arms, as well as some tingling or numbness of the fingers.

Of all the changes that occur in a woman who has become pregnant, the most subtle are those in the hematologic (blood) system. The amount of blood in circulation increases markedly (up to 50 percent) during pregnancy. This increase begins in the first trimester and accelerates rapidly in the second trimester. It begins to slow in the last weeks of pregnancy. This dramatic increase in blood volume is vitally important because the body needs to meet the increasing nutritional needs of the growing fetus and enlarging uterus. It also protects the mother from excessive blood loss, which may occur during or after delivery.

Nutrition

Many questions arise during pregnancy about what to eat, how much to eat, and how much weight to gain. It has long been recognized that pregnant women can maintain a balanced diet by regularly choosing foods from the well-known four basic food groups. A pregnant woman should follow these diet guidelines:

1. *Meat, fish, poultry, and eggs*: three or more servings a day. *Never* eat uncooked meat or raw fish or seafood.
2. *Fruits and vegetables*: four or more servings a day.
3. *Milk, milk products, and cheese*: four or more servings a day.
4. *Whole grain or enriched bread or cereal*: four or more servings a day.

Vegetarians and vegans (those who eat no meat, eggs, or milk) will have to work harder and be more careful about their diets to make sure that they get enough proteins, vitamins A, B_{12}, and D, iron, and calcium. Vitamins and mineral supplements may be recommended.

Pregnant women should be careful to avoid foods that tend to worsen problems associated with pregnancy. Salt promotes swelling, so canned foods and processed foods, which usually contain a lot of salt, should be avoided. Sodas and other foods high in sugar are low in nutrients and contribute to excessive weight gain, so pregnant women should eliminate or reduce their intake of these substances. Fried, fatty foods and greasy foods can cause heartburn, gas, and constipation, as well as aggravate existing gallbladder problems.

The recommendations for weight gain during pregnancy have changed considerably over the past thirty years. Research focusing on the relationship between a woman's adequate weight gain and the well-being of her pregnancy shows that desirable weight gain during pregnancy is related to weight *before* pregnancy. That is, there is no longer an ideal that governs all women. The current recommendations take into account a woman's prepregnancy weight and height. As recommended in *Nutrition During Pregnancy*, published by the National Academy of Science in 1990, a woman who starts her pregnancy within an optimal weight range for her height should gain a total amount of about twenty-five to thirty-five pounds. This allows for a gain of three and one-half pounds during the first trimester and one pound a week for the remainder of the pregnancy. A woman who is underweight for her height at the start of pregnancy can tolerate a weight gain of twenty-eight to forty pounds, depending largely on the degree to which she is underweight before her pregnancy begins. This works out to a five-pound weight gain during the first trimester and slightly more than a one-pound weight gain per week for the remainder of the pregnancy. A woman who is overweight at the start of her pregnancy may need to keep her total weight gain to as little as fifteen to twenty-five pounds, starting with a two-pound weight gain during the first trimester and adding two-thirds pound per week for the remainder of the pregnancy.

Excessive weight gain is undesirable, but a pregnant woman should never attempt to lose weight by dieting. Insufficient weight gain and poor nutrition during pregnancy can have devastating and lasting effects on a baby, both before and after birth. Whenever possible, a woman should discuss her questions about nutrition and weight during pregnancy with her doctor before her pregnancy begins. Planning and preparing for pregnancy can increase the chances of having a happy and successful outcome.

Labor and Delivery

The process of labor and delivery is truly amazing and still little understood. We do know that there is a relationship between the size and the position of the baby. There is also a relationship between the width of the pelvic bones and the strength of the contractions that open (or dilate) the cervix and push the baby out. Traditionally, these factors have been referred to as the "passenger," the "passage," and the "powers." Although we do not really know what causes labor to begin under normal circumstances, it is well understood that contractions must be both strong and regular to dilate the cervix as well as to push the baby down and out.

The size and position of the passenger are as important as is the adequacy of the contractions. A baby that is not in the correct position or that is too big will not pass through the pelvis, no matter how strong or frequent the contractions. The ideal position for the baby to be in just prior to birth is head-first, with the top of the head pointing down toward the vagina. This position occurs in 90 percent of pregnancies. Approximately 2 percent of the time the baby is positioned bottom-first, or breech. Your physician can make a simple examination (called Leopold maneuvers) after thirty-five weeks of pregnancy to try to determine if your baby is head-first. If there is a question about the position of the fetus, an *ultrasound* can be done, using sound waves to "look inside" the body and see the baby. Although ultrasound may be useful, it does have a considerable margin of error when considering fetal weight; thus estimates of fetal weight (the size of the fetus) are not entirely accurate and are difficult to obtain using ultrasound.

Vaginal birth is clearly the preferred route of delivery and it occurs a majority of the time, but cesarean section (c-section) is sometimes a necessary alternative. A c-section requires a surgical incision through a pregnant woman's skin, muscles of the abdominal wall, and uterus. The baby is delivered through the incision, and once the placenta is delivered, the uterus, abdominal wall, and skin are sutured closed.

There are three common circumstances in which c-sections are performed. *Fetal distress,* usually diagnosed during labor, is a sign that indicates that the fetus is not tolerating labor well and may be in jeopardy if labor continues much longer. In this situation, the c-section is performed as quickly as possible. (Fetal distress may also be diagnosed *before* labor begins and is also an indication for c-section.) Another circumstance requiring a c-section occurs when labor is progressing abnormally but there is no fetal distress. This may be known as *failure to progress,* or as *dysfunctional labor.* In these situations, the cesarean is done after labor has been under way for some time and after steps have been taken to increase the chances of vaginal delivery.

The third common reason for doing a c-section occurs when the woman has already had a c-section in the past. For the majority of women, only those who have had classical c-sections are *required* to have cesarean deliveries for all subsequent pregnancies. Classical c-sections are done infrequently in obstetrics today. Most c-sections involve making a *low-transverse* incision in the uterus, which enables a woman to be a candidate for a trial of labor for vaginal birth after cesarean (VBAC). VBAC is being discussed and encouraged more often as one of the ways to decrease the number of cesarean deliveries being done. Cesareans require anesthesia, and because c-sections increase the risk of infection and surgical complications, doctors try to limit doing them to times when they are absolutely necessary.

Anesthesia is often used in vaginal deliveries as well. There are several types of anesthesia available for women who are about to give birth. An *epidural* anesthetic is usually given when active labor has been established. When it is working properly, it eliminates the discomfort of the contractions but does not stop them or slow labor. This medication allows the patient to be more comfortable while her labor continues.

The *subarachnoid block* ("spinal") is an anesthetic that produces complete loss of feeling below the level of the spinal cord into which it is injected. It will stop contractions from occurring. For this reason it is not given until the end of labor, just before vaginal delivery is about to occur. When a subarachnoid block is used as an anesthetic, it is necessary to assist the delivery of the baby's head, using either forceps or a vacuum extractor, because the delivering mother will not be able to push the baby out. Spinals and epidurals may also be used during c-sections.

The most common analgesic used in labor is demerol, a narcotic medication given in small amounts after labor has been well established, either as an intramuscular (IM) injection or through intravenous (IV) tubing. Demerol helps to relieve some of the pain of the contractions and relax the mother so that she can rest between them. Being more relaxed may help a woman's labor progress.

Two points about analgesia and anesthesia must be made very clear: First, no woman in labor should be given any medication unless she requests it, and second, requesting medication for relief during labor is not an admission of failure. Labor can be long and hard. Pain relief during labor is intended to help make both a physically and emotionally demanding process easier to tolerate. It should not be considered unreasonable to request some comfort and relief when medications are safe and available and can make the quality of the experience better. If you have questions about the use of pain medications in labor, do not hesitate to ask your obstetrician-gynecologist. Do not be distracted by narrow and restrictive ideas of what is expected during labor. The use of pain medication is a very personal decision. Your doctor can help you to decide if you wish to use anesthesia or analgesics, but only you know the amount of pain you can tolerate.

Postdelivery Changes

There are a number of physical changes that occur in a woman's body in the *postpartum* period, that is, the first six weeks after delivery. The breasts remain large and produce milk if the child is being breastfed. The breasts get smaller if the new mother is not breastfeeding. The uterus gradually returns to its normal size, and there is a general weight loss. In fact, almost all of the changes caused by the pregnancy will be reversed, but some, such as darkening of the skin, may not go away quickly, if at all. Remember that it took nine months for all of these changes to occur. Thus women who have just gone through pregnancy must realize that the changes to their bodies will not go away in one week or even one month after delivery.

The emotional changes that women experience postpartum can be dramatic. There are the obvious feelings of joy and elation that the pregnancy is over and all is well. There may also be feelings of anxiety and apprehension that come with the realization of the new responsibilities and work involved with the care of the newborn. These are normal feelings that usually pass quickly. Postpartum blues or postpartum depression, which is well recognizedl and extensively written about, is experienced by some women. The cause of this problem remains unknown. It should go away on its own. Nevertheless, it is important for women to have good support systems at this time. If the depression does not go away within a reasonable amount of time, psychiatric evaluation should be considered without delay.

About the Author

Dr. Richard Henderson received his medical degree from Howard University College of Medicine. He completed his residency in obstetrics and gynecology at the Medical Center of Delaware and is a fellow of the American College of Obstetricians and Gynecologists.

Dr. Henderson is in private practice in Wilmington, Delaware. He was president of the Obstetrical and Gynecology Society of Delaware from 1993 to 1994 and has served in numerous posts as an advocate of women's health care.

QUESTIONS FOR THE DOCTOR

Q: *I have heard that if someone is diagnosed with diabetes during pregnancy it can predict the return of diabetes in later life. Is this true?*

A: One of the complex changes that can occur in a woman's body during pregnancy is new onset diabetes, or *gestational diabetes*. It usually goes away within six weeks of delivery. If a woman develops gestational diabetes, there is an increased risk that she may develop diabetes later in life, but this cannot be predicted with certainty. A woman who has gestational diabetes should be tested for true diabetes six or more weeks after delivery. If a woman has known diabetes, it is very important that she discuss pregnancy with her obstetrician/gynecologist before becoming pregnant. The diabetic woman should also notify her ob/gyn as soon as pregnancy is diagnosed so that prenatal care may be started without delay. Uncontrolled diabetes during pregnancy has been associated with serious fetal birth defects and can also be fatal to the mother.

Q: *I have two children. When I was last pregnant I was told that I had high blood pressure in the final three weeks of the pregnancy. Should I be concerned?*

A: High blood pressure that develops at any time during pregnancy is a reason for concern. If hypertension is present before pregnancy and is uncontrolled, there can be very serious side effects for both the mother and her fetus. In fact, if allowed to continue throughout pregnancy, it can be deadly. Therefore, it is crucial that a woman with hypertension have both early and consistent prenatal care for her high-risk pregnancy.

When hypertension develops as a result of changes caused by the pregnancy, it is called *pre-eclampsia* or *pregnancy-induced hypertension* (PIH). Pre-eclampsia also places both the mother and fetus at risk for a poor outcome and must be followed very closely. The hypertension associated with the pre-eclampsia usually goes away within six weeks after delivery and does not require any additional treatment.

Q: *I am seven months pregnant and I've been noticing that I have occasional spots of blood in my underwear. Should I be concerned?*

A: Bleeding at any time during pregnancy should be investigated, and you should not hesitate to call your doctor. A single exam with a speculum can determine if the bleeding is coming from the walls of the vagina or the outside of the cervix, as may occur after sexual intercourse or if infections such as yeast or trichomonas are present. If it appears that the bleeding may be coming from outside the uterus, hospitalization for bedrest and further evaluation may be recommended. An ultrasound test is very useful in this situation to locate and evaluate the placenta and the fetus.

Q: *My husband and I are trying to become pregnant. I have a serious amount of sinus congestion and I occasionally take over-the-counter sinus medications. Can I continue taking these medications while I'm pregnant?*

A: The general recommendation is to avoid all medications in the first twelve weeks of pregnancy unless they have been discussed with a doctor first. Remember, all of the major organ systems are formed in the fetus in the first twelve weeks. Some medications are known to cause problems, but there are many more that we have no idea about: hence the recommendation to avoid medication in the first twelve weeks if possible. If you are on prescribed medication for any condition, inform your obstetrician and the doctor who prescribed the medication as soon as the pregnancy is diagnosed.

Q: *I always hear about ultrasound tests used in pregnancy. Can they hurt the baby?*
A: There is no evidence that use of ultrasound can hurt your baby. Ultrasound uses sound waves, not X rays, to obtain a picture of where the baby is, how big it is, or where the placenta is located. It is a very valuable tool when used appropriately. Use of ultrasound merely to try to determine the sex of the fetus is inappropriate.

Q: *What is an ectopic pregnancy?*
A: An ectopic, or tubal, pregnancy occurs when the fertilized egg or developing embryo implants itself outside the uterus. Most commonly (more than 95 percent of the time), ectopic pregnancies occur in the Fallopian tube—hence the name "tubal" pregnancy. Other places ectopic pregnancies may occur include the ovary, the cervix, or the abdominal cavity. Ectopic pregnancies occur when the Fallopian tube is partially blocked, preventing the developing embryo from entering the uterus. If a tubal pregnancy is untreated, it may rupture the Fallopian tube and lead to internal bleeding that could be life threatening. Therefore, when a diagnosis of ectopic pregnancy is made, either surgery or other medical management should be initiated without delay.

Q: *How many weeks can a woman stay pregnant and have a healthy baby?*
A: Most physicians encourage delivery by the end of forty-two weeks of gestation. Sometimes this time is prolonged, say, if the mother has not sought prenatal care from a physician and simply arrives at the hospital when she is already in labor or stays at home for delivery. The danger for a long-term baby is that the placenta may not supply the fetus with blood containing sufficient oxygen, and the life of the baby might be threatened. You should always see your health care provider on a regular basis during pregnancy.

Q: *What do you think of nurse-midwives? Do you think they would be helpful in delivering children?*
A: Clearly nurses or midwives can do a wonderful job delivering children; in fact, they provide one of the many options for delivery available to women. It is most important, no matter whom you have chosen to be your health care provider, to have care throughout pregnancy,

from the very beginning, and to be provided with an environment for delivery that is safe, clean, and readily accessible in case you have an emergency. You should discuss these issues with your partner and with appropriate health professionals in your area. Talk to other parents. Find out about their experiences with different physicians and different health care workers and determine what will work best for you. This is a happy time in your life, and it is also an extremely important one. You need to give your baby the opportunity to be as healthy as he or she can be.

12

Prostate Cancer and Other Urologic Problems

Walter L. Gerber, M.D., F.A.C.S.

The prostate is a small, pecan-sized gland that is located under the bladder only in males. If the bottom half of the bladder is visualized as a funnel, the prostate gland surrounds the stem of the funnel just after it narrows. The stem, called the *urethra,* drains the urine through the penis. The back half of the prostate can be felt by your doctor when he does a rectal examination, since the prostate is only a fraction of an inch away.

Normally, the prostate supplies over half of the liquid that comes from the tip of the penis when a man has sex and ejaculates; this fluid nourishes the sperm and provides materials they need to fertilize an egg. The prostate also helps to keep men from leaking their urine by providing support to the urethra. In addition, the prostate seems to play a role in preventing bladder infections because of the high levels it contains of the mineral zinc.

Prostate Enlargement

Of men over age fifty, 75 percent will have some symptoms of prostatic enlargement in their lifetimes and 20 percent will require therapy by the time they reach age eighty. The gland may reach the size of a golf ball or even a tangerine. It is important to remember that prostate enlargement does *not* mean that cancer is present. Although cancer can occur in men with enlarged prostates, there is no direct link; however, this does not

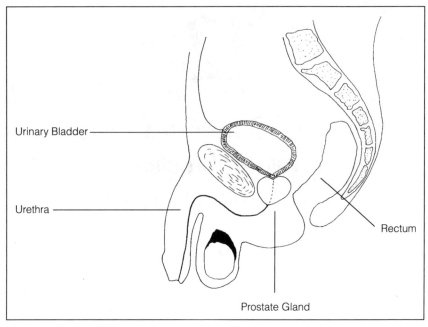

Urinary Bladder

Urethra

Rectum

Prostate Gland

The Prostate and Surrounding Structures

mean that benign (or noncancerous) prostatic enlargement should be ignored.

The manifestations of an enlarged prostate can vary widely over time. They are often influenced by other health and situational problems that affect a person's life. In general, doctors divide the symptoms from benign enlargement of the prostate (*benign prostatic hypertrophy,* or BPH) into obstructive and irritative problems. *Obstructive* disturbances include a decreased force to the urinary stream, hesitancy, incomplete bladder emptying, a need to strain to void, and postvoid dribbling. *Irritative* complaints (caused by bladder instability) include frequency of urination, voiding in small volumes, urgency, urination at night, and even pain during urination. Over half of the men who have enlarged prostates describe both obstructive and irritative difficulties.

Put more simply, if you can no longer "write your name in the snow," you may have a problem with the urinary stream. If you find that you are waking up two or three times a night to go to the bathroom or the need to urinate is disturbing your sleep pattern, if you have to lean forward as you urinate, or if your pants are wet after you finish, your prostate may be enlarged.

Why is it so important to treat prostate and urologic problems? Certainly, the inconvenience of not being able to urinate effectively and efficiently, as well as the embarrassment these conditions may cause, is enough to prompt you to seek medical attention. But from a medical standpoint, men who have trouble with their prostate gland are at risk for infections of the bladder and kidneys and even the complete, sudden, and painful inability to urinate at all.

Another way to picture the prostate is to think of it as a hard-boiled egg with a straw running through it. The straw (or stem of the funnel) is the urethra. When the prostate enlarges in the absence of cancer, the yolk of the egg squeezes on the urethra, making it more difficult to pass urine. Because of the partial blockage, urine may build up in the bladder, and you can urinate only when the pressure builds to a sufficient point to force urine through the constricted "straw."

There are many things that can be done to help alleviate the problem of an enlarged prostate. *Prostatectomy*, surgery that is usually performed through the urethra with very small instruments or even a laser, is currently the most widely accepted treatment for blockage caused by an enlarged prostate. The "yolk" of the hard-boiled egg is scraped out in small pieces, enlarging the channel through which the urine flows. The "white" and the "shell" of the egg are not removed. This procedure is called a *trans-* ("through") *urethral removal of the prostate*, or TURP.

It must be remembered that a TURP does not remove the entire prostate; only the center of the gland is eliminated. Rectal examinations to detect cancer developing in the "white" of the egg are still needed.

Surgery is usually successful, even for patients of advanced age. But there are risks, including the normal risks of surgery as well as the risk of impotence. More than four hundred thousand TURPs are performed each year in the United States; the cumulative cost exceeds one billion dollars. This figure does not include the cost of diagnosis, time lost from work, or nonsurgical therapies for complications such as urinary infections. As our population ages, an even greater number of men may ultimately require some form of prostatic treatment. Because of the risks and expenses of surgery, alternatives are being sought. Experimentally, balloons have been developed that can be inflated inside the portion of the urethra that runs through the prostate; the channel expands, cracks the "yolk," and leaves the "straw" less obstructed than before. Alternatively, a *stent*, a spiral tube like the spring in a ballpoint pen, can be placed inside the urethra; its fairly rigid walls hold the channel open and allow urine to pass more freely. A promising new treatment involves heating the prostate gland using energy similar to that from a microwave oven; the power is applied either through the urethra or through the rectum. The heated prostate seems to shrink.

Several new medications are now available that can help reduce the size of the prostate. The most widely known is Proscar. It blocks the formation of the active form of testosterone, the major male sex hormone, which is needed by the prostate to maintain its growth. A disadvantage of this type of drug is that it must be taken for many years to prevent regrowth of the prostate. In addition, the drug interferes with a blood test to help detect early cancer in the prostate. Other drugs, called *alpha-adrenergic "blocking" agents*, have been shown to help relax microscopic muscle fibers within the prostate and the opening of the bladder, increasing urine flow. Interestingly, these drugs were originally developed to fight high blood pressure.

Prostate Cancer

To repeat, if you have an enlarged prostate, this does not mean that you have or will develop prostate cancer. Nevertheless, *adenocarcinoma of the prostate* has now become the second most common cause of death in adult men and the most common malignancy in American men over age seventy. Seventeen percent of all new malignancies discovered in males, and 10 percent of all cancer deaths in males, are because of this disease. The American Cancer Society has estimated that there will be one hundred thousand new cases of prostate cancer diagnosed each year and that more than thirty thousand men will die from their disease. As with most malignancies, the cause is obscure; however, genetic factors, hormonal influences, and chemical carcinogens may all play roles. A relationship to venereal disease has been proposed but has never been proven.

Cancer of the prostate may be completely silent until the tumor has become large enough to cause obstruction of the flow of urine. Urologic surgeons typically find 10 percent to 15 percent of all cancers of the prostate when they perform a TURP for what they thought was benign prostatic enlargement. These patients may be lucky, because their cancer is often discovered early enough for effective treatment. Unfortunately, a large percentage of patients do not seek medical attention until they notice symptoms caused by spread of the cancer throughout the body.

The thought of cancer is frightening, but there are ways to detect prostatic cancer early. Rectal examination is still the least expensive and best method available. Many cancers show a more generalized pattern rather than a discrete lump, however, and these are more difficult to detect by rectal examination. In addition, the rectal examination allows the doctor to feel only the "back" portion of the prostate gland.

The best hope for early detection of prostate cancer seems to lie in the combination of a rectal examination and a simple blood test for a "tumor marker," a substance in the blood caused by the presence of a cancer. The most sensitive and specific tumor marker at the present time is prostatic specific antigen (PSA). Low PSA levels correlate well with a low incidence of malignancy; high levels also correlate well with a high probability that cancer is present. An exciting discovery is that mildly elevated PSA levels seem to correlate with a significant chance that a cancer is present but is confined to the prostate; thus it is more easily curable with existing methods of treatment.

The efficacy of testing PSA levels as a screening tool for prostate cancer in the general population strongly justifies its use; its benefits outweigh its costs. The combination of PSA and rectal examination is critical to early detection and treatment of prostate cancer. Neither an abnormal rectal exam nor a higher than normal PSA test proves that a cancer is present, however: they are only warnings. When a physician is concerned about the possible presence of a cancer, a biopsy of the prostate is needed. This almost painless procedure is often combined with an ultrasound of the prostate and is performed through the rectum, since cancers usually begin in the "white" of the hard-boiled egg and do not grow centrally toward the urethra until more advanced.

If prostate cancer is caught early, cure is possible with major surgery or radiation so long as the tumor remains within the capsule of the prostate (the "shell" of the hard-boiled egg). As the malignancy spreads to other parts of the body, it becomes more difficult to treat, and the success rate decreases. Important new developments in CAT scans, MRI exams, and even "belly button" surgery with the laparoscope have begun to make diagnosis easier. Treatment is tailored to the individual and to the extent of his disease.

Infertility

Of course, a problem with the prostate is not the only urologic condition that men face. *Infertility* has been defined as the inability to produce a living child after one year of unprotected intercourse. This cold, clinical definition does little to describe the suffering and emotional upheaval that an infertile couple experiences.

Recent statistics suggest that nearly one out of every six couples (15 percent) are unable to conceive a child within a year; another 10 percent experience difficulty when they attempt to have a second or third child. Thus, 25 percent of all couples will need fertility testing and counseling. Male factors will be responsible in 50 percent of cases: 25 percent of the time alone and 25 percent of the time combined with problems related to the female partner. Clearly, it is important that both partners be evaluated for infertility, but this chapter stresses problems related to the male.

To begin to determine the cause, physicians must identify and eliminate practices that may decrease fertility, especially in patients with marginal semen quality. This requires a thorough medical and sexual history. In some instances, simple remedies may be all that are needed to resolve the problem, such as better timing of sex. Men who ejaculate every day may not be allowing enough time to replenish their supplies of active sperm. Conversely, sperm may age inside men if intercourse is infrequent, yielding sperm of decreased quality. "Saving up" the sperm until the right moment is not effective.

The patient's use of medications and drugs also needs to be evaluated. There is some evidence that marijuana decreases male hormone levels, lowers the total number of sperm, decreases the ability of sperm to swim, and increases the chances for abnormal-appearing sperm. Caffeine and alcohol may also be harmful.

A careful physical examination is mandatory. Certainly, abnormal testes, whatever the cause, need to be recognized, even if no remedy can be proposed. The man may have a condition called *hypospadias*. This is an abnormality of the penis in which the urethra opens underneath the penis and not at the tip. Individuals with this condition may have fertility problems because the sperm have difficulty reaching the vagina. Sperm collected from these men can easily be used to get their partners pregnant through artificial insemination.

Examination of the semen, produced by masturbation, is the most important diagnostic test of the infertile male. Most of the sperm are found in the fluid that comes out first; poor collections that miss this first portion may yield information that is useless or incorrect. For the purpose of this test, therefore, the man should attempt to maximize the quality and number of sperm. For example, he should not ejaculate for three or four days before the sample collection. Sperm do not tolerate low temperatures well, and the semen should not be exposed to outside conditions, which is the reason the patient may be asked to produce a specimen in the doctor's office. Despite the embarrassment, this is important. Whenever possible, the semen analysis should be scheduled for those times when the man's partner is not making eggs, perhaps even when she is menstruating. In this way, sperm will not be "wasted."

Many different aspects of the sperm need to be evaluated. A normal semen specimen has a volume of one-half to one teaspoon, although small variations in volume are probably not significant. The ejaculate should coagulate almost immediately and then should reliquify within fifteen to twenty minutes (in order to observe this, the semen has to be examined as quickly as possible after ejaculation). The sperm concentration should be greater than 20 million/cc, and the total number of sperm must be greater than 100 million for the count to be normal. At least 75 percent of the sperm should be alive, and 60 percent to 65 percent should be swimming normally. The quality and appearance of the sperm are as important as the numbers.

If the first semen analysis is normal, further testing of the man may be delayed until the woman's initial evaluation has been completed. Of course, certain life-style changes may be recommended to the man at the first visit even if his semen appears normal. For example, decreasing caffeine and alcohol consumption and stopping the use of baths and the wearing of jockey shorts may be advised. Experts disagree as to the importance of elevated testicular temperatures caused by hot baths or tight underwear. Perhaps slightly elevated temperatures are more significant in decreasing fertility among patients wiith borderline semen quality than they are among normal men. In any event, these changes in life-style are relatively easy and should be tried early.

If the initial semen analysis is abnormal, additional semen tests should be performed at least several weeks apart. This delay allows for the passage of time to correct any temporary problems. Simple stresses, such as a fever or even extensive driving during a vacation, can produce temporary abnormalities. Men with borderline or marginal fertility may be more susceptible to such mild outside forces.

Testicular failure of varying degrees is the most common cause of decreased male fertility. An oral medication, *clomiphene citrate,* has been of value in some patients with low sperm counts. The drug is thought to work by fooling the brain into thinking that the testosterone level is low, causing the release of hormones that stimulate the testicles. Even though the medicine is prescribed widely by fertility specialists, the Food and Drug Administration has not given approval for its use in men, and patients must be informed of this.

The most important treatable cause of infertility in men is a *varicocele*. In this condition, veins draining blood out of the testes have malfunctioning valves that cause them to become much larger than normal. Large varicoceles may be visible when the patient stands upright; they can be felt easily but should disappear completely when the man lies down. The testis on the affected side is often smaller than its mate. Small varicoceles may be more difficult for the doctor to detect, but the size of a varicocele is not important, only its presence.

Varicoceles are found in approximately 40 percent of men seen by an infertility specialist. Although the cause of this abnormality and the ways it may interfere with semen quality are not known, it can be treated with surgery. Perhaps the availability of laparoscopic ("belly button") surgery will make it easier for the patient to decide to have the abnormal venous drainage repaired. Pregnancy rates after elimination of varicoceles are as high as 50 percent to 60 percent, even in couples who have not been successful at becoming pregnant for many years.

With continued improvements in artificial insemination and in vitro fertilization techniques, an increased number of couples will be able to achieve a pregnancy, even when the man has very low numbers of sperm. The knowledge that new treatments are available should give hope to many individuals that they will be able to become parents.

Impotence

Infertility is not the male's only sexual problem. More than ten million adult males have complaints about obtaining or maintaining erections. If good communication is present between partners, satisfactory sex may still be possible, even if the man's erections are diminished. A man can ejaculate without an erection, since the processes that cause the two phenomena are completely independent.

As we learn more about how erections take place, we can be more successful at identifying specific causes of decreased performance. Doctors no longer assume that psychological problems cause most of the difficulties. Many medications, for example, are known to affect erectile capability, especially those used to treat high blood pressure and heart disease. These drugs must be continued because of their importance in treating much more life-threatening conditions; however, it may be possible to change to an equally effective medication that causes fewer side effects related to erections.

Erections take place through a complicated process involving nerves, muscles, blood vessels, and hormones. Nerve impulses from the brain relax microscopic muscles that surround the arteries that bring blood into the penis as well as the blood channels within the penis. When these muscles relax, blood can then flow into and become trapped within the penis, making it hard.

The major cause of diminished blood inflow or failure to fill the penis adequately is *atherosclerotic vascular disease* (hardening of the arteries). This tends to be diffuse and is associated with a history of vascular risk factors, including smoking and diabetes. Surgery to bring new blood to the penis has not met with as much success in the United States as it has in Europe. Failure to store blood in the penis for a sufficiently long period, called *venous leak,* is also most commonly attributed to factors such as diabetes, high levels of cholesterol, hypertension, and cigarette smoking. Surgery to tie off veins, in order to trap blood more effectively in the penis, is not popular among most urologists and vascular surgeons in the United States.

The current gold standard of therapy is the *penile prosthesis,* which is a type of implant placed completely inside the penis to give enough rigidity to allow for intercourse. Some implants cause a permanent erection; others are hydraulically inflated when an erection is desired. A wide variety of styles and models from a number of manufacturers is available. The complications and failures of many of these mechanical devices are significant, however, and not all patients are suitable candidates.

Some men cannot obtain an erection because of abnormal neurologic responses. The major diseases causing this condition include multiple sclerosis, radical pelvic surgery, and spinal cord injury. Patients can be taught to inject medicines that bypass the defective nerves directly into the side of the penis. These self-injections are being used successfully with minimal discomfort and few complications.

Couples must be reminded that there is more to love than sex and more to sex than vaginal penetration. Sex therapy and psychological counseling should be a part of any treatment program, even in the presence of known organic disease.

About the Author

Dr. Walter L. Gerber is a graduate of Princeton University and the Albert Einstein College of Medicine in New York. He received his surgical training at Johns Hopkins University and his urologic specialty training at the Washington University of St. Louis. He also performed basic medical research for two years at the National Institutes of Health in Bethesda, Maryland.

After teaching full time at the University of Iowa School of Medicine for eight years, he moved to Philadelphia and taught full time at Temple University School of Medicine. Dr. Gerber is now in private practice at the Albert Einstein Medical Center in Philadelphia. He is also an associate professor of urology and of obstetrics and gynecology at Temple University School of Medicine.

Dr. Gerber is licensed to practice medicine in six states. He is a member of more than twenty local, national, and international medical organizations and is the immediate past president of the Philadelphia Urological Association, one of the oldest specialty societies in the United States. He is a Distinguished Lecturer for the American Cancer Society and the author of more than forty-five publications.

QUESTIONS FOR THE DOCTOR

Q: *What are the warning signs of bladder cancer?*

A: *Bladder cancer* can occur in both men and women. Tumors of the bladder are the second most common of all tumors of the genitourinary system. In fact, in men the rate of bladder cancer is second only to that of prostate cancer. Seventy-five percent of all tumors of the bladder are found in men. The number of cases of bladder cancer in women seems to be rising as they increasingly smoke and work in dirty places.

Most bladder cancers are seen in patients older than age fifty. The tumors are produced by a combination of two factors: a cancer-causing agent in the urine and a susceptibility to that agent. A host of chemicals found in people who work, for example, in the rubber, chemical, and leather industries have been shown to produce bladder cancer in animals and have been implicated in human cancers as well. There is concern that a naturally and commonly occurring chemical in our own bodies may be altered by smoking and can then lead to bladder cancer.

Blood in the urine is the most common finding in bladder cancer. The bleeding can occur off and on without other symptoms and may sometimes be in such small quantities that it can be detected only by looking at the urine through a microscope. Pain and burning with urination may be present and may be confused with a simple bladder infection.

The prognosis or outcome from bladder cancer depends mainly on the stage of the tumor, which reflects the amount of invasion by the tumor through the wall of the bladder. Obviously, the deeper the cancer goes, the greater the chance it will spread to other sites and be harder to cure. As with other forms of cancer, it is important to detect bladder cancer early.

Q: *I am concerned about testicular cancer.*
A: Each year more than six thousand men, usually between the ages of twenty and thirty-five, are found to have *testicular cancer.* Whites are affected more than African Americans. It is a very serious condition, but most patients can be completely cured if the disease is detected early. The most significant risk factor is an undescended or poorly descended testicle or one previously affected by mumps; however, the tumor may develop in what previously seemed to be a normal testis.

Initial signs of the disease are few. Most patients seek attention because they have a painless lump or swelling in one testis. Testicular pain, discomfort on urination, and other complaints are not common. Because of the lack of discomfort, many men delay seeing their doctor longer than they should. Others delay because they are embarrassed or because they are afraid that a cancer will actually be found.

If testicular cancer is suspected, the painless test of ultrasound can be done to evaluate the problem. If a cancer is present, surgery to remove the testicle must be performed because the cancer can spread dramatically if it is missed. It is important to remember that a man can still have normal erections and be able to produce children with only one functioning testicle.

If a man does a testicular self-examination every month, he can detect abnormal lumps early. If the disease is caught quickly, life expectancy is great. If you are interested in more information, the American Cancer Society has free pamphlets available.

Q: *We want to have our baby circumcised, but our insurance won't pay. What should we do?*
A: In the current era of cost-cutting in medicine, circumcision is considered by many to be an elective, cosmetic procedure. This is clearly an individual choice for a family to make, and in certain cultures it is

a religious choice. There is some evidence that bladder infections are more common in uncircumcised infants and children than in those who are circumcised. Cancer of the penis, although uncommon, is almost never seen in a man who was circumcised at birth. The advantage of circumcision is that it is far easier to keep the penis clean; but if a man practices good hygiene, there is no reason to think he cannot achieve the same cleanliness without a circumcision.

If you are going to pay for a circumcision yourself, be aware that prices can range anywhere from $500 to $6,000, depending on who performs the procedure, what facilities are used, and whether or not an operating room is required. In general, the older the child, the greater the chance that your doctor will want to have him under a general anesthetic.

Q: Is male birth control available?
A: Yes, in two forms: condoms and vasectomy, which is permanent. Some studies indicate that a hormone pill for men may be available in the future.

Q: I'm a thirty-seven-year-old male, and I have had two urinary tract infections in the past year. Should I be concerned?
A: Yes, you do need to be evaluated since urinary tract infections in males are far less common than in females. You should have a physical examination that includes a rectal exam to check your prostate. You will need a bacterial test of your urine. In your case, a simple infection in the prostate is most likely. More serious kidney or bladder problems may be present, however. Other tests, such as an X ray that shows the kidneys and the tubes that connect them to the bladder, and even a check to see if you have a stricture in the urethra (the channel that carries urine through the penis), may be needed.

Q: I am in my late seventies and am married to a thirty-five-year-old woman. Can I still have children?
A: Many men at your age are still able to father children. A semen analysis can give you an idea of your fertility potential if you wish. You and your partner should consider the social consequences of your fathering a child late in life and discuss your concerns with your health care providers.

Q: I never had problems with my sex life until recently, when I began taking a blood pressure pill. I am having trouble achieving erections. Could it be because my blood pressure is lower? Should I stop my medicine?

A: Bringing your blood pressure into the normal range does not usually cause problems with erections. The medicine itself, however, could produce erectile disturbances as a side effect. One group of drugs in particular, called *beta-blockers,* has been linked to impotence. Since treating your high blood pressure is so necessary, it is very important that you not discontinue your medicine. Talk to your doctor; there are many choices available and a slightly different drug might be right for you.

Q: *I have heard that the best way to manage prostate cancer is to watch it carefully and not do invasive surgery right away. What do you think?*

A: Prostate cancer affects men of many different ages and varies widely in the amount of cancer that is present. Treatment needs to be individualized, and no two patients are exactly alike. It may make sense for you and your doctor to watch a small cancer if you are, say, age seventy-five, but not to watch the same cancer if you are age sixty. Surgery may need to be done early so as not to miss an opportunity to cure a patient. Not all cancers require major surgery or radiation therapy, however. If you are diagnosed with prostate cancer, you and your urologist need to examine all of the facts and test results, agree on a plan, and review the treatment periodically.

13

Sinusitis and Allergies

Max Ronis, M.D.

An estimated thirty million people in the United States suffer from sinus disease. It is further estimated that approximately one-third of all patients who come to pediatricians and primary care doctors have a complaint that refers either to the upper respiratory tract (nose, sinuses, or throat) or to the ears. In order to understand the problems that can arise within the nose and sinuses and to appreciate the method by which these problems are approached, it is very important to know a little about the anatomy and the function of both the sinus and the nasal cavities.

The Nose

The external nose is formed by bone, cartilage, and soft tissue. It is just a projection that has very little to do with the airway and breathing. The various sizes and shapes of the external nose are determined by many factors, including racial characteristics, genetics, and familial traits.

The inside of the nose is the functional portion. It is divided into two separate nasal cavities by a bony and cartilaginous structure called the *nasal septum* that more or less runs down the center of the nose. On either side of the nasal cavity there are little tufts of tissue called *turbinates* that function to warm, humidify, and filter the air we breathe. The mucous membrane that covers these turbinates has an extremely rich blood supply. These tissues can swell and become very engorged under

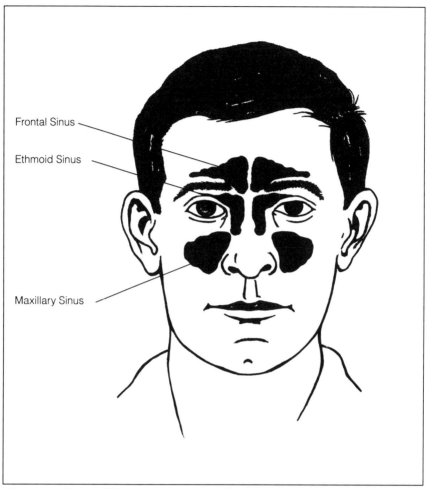

Frontal Sinus

Ethmoid Sinus

Maxillary Sinus

View of the Frontal, Ethmoid, and Maxillary Sinuses

certain conditions having to do with infections and allergies, and the nasal mucus membrane that lines the nose is designed specifically to do so. Higher up, along the roof of the nose there are specialized nerve cells called *olfactory cells*, where the sense of smell is determined. Smell (or olfaction) aids in the sense of taste. Other than the tastes of salt, sour, sweet, and bitter, everything we taste is mediated and controlled by the sense of olfaction, and much of what we detect in the environment is also. That is why the nose plays such an important role in our day-to-day activities.

The Sinuses and Their Function

Surrounding the nasal cavity and the eyes are four sets of air-containing spaces called *paranasal sinuses*. Starting in childhood, they become filled with air and grow; they reach their full size by adolescence.

The *frontal sinuses* are located above the eyes, just above the eyebrows, and meet in the midline. They are usually of unequal size and are shaped like an irregular pyramid, pointing upward. About 15 percent of adults may have only one frontal sinus, and about 5 percent to 10 percent may have no frontal sinuses at all. However, no functional problems result from the absence of these sinuses. The *maxillary sinuses* are under the eye and lie beneath the cheek. Both the maxillary sinuses and the frontal sinuses drain into the nose.

Between the eyes, the *ethmoid sinuses* are located on each side at the root of the nose. These multiple, thin-walled sinus spaces are filled with air. Finally, in the middle of the head, behind the nose and the eyes, are the *sphenoid sinuses,* which can vary greatly in size and shape. The pituitary gland, which controls hormonal function, sits above and slightly behind the sphenoid sinuses.

Medical science does not have a complete picture of sinus function. We do know that all of the sinuses have small openings that drain into the nose. The sinuses are thought to provide the following functions:

- They lighten the weight of the skull by substituting air-containing spaces for solid bone
- They provide a protection by lessening potential impact on adjacent vital structures, such as the brain and the eyes
- They act as a resonating chamber for voice production
- They also act as an insulator or a temperature control mechanism for the structures they surround

Mucous Membrane Irritation

Normally, the mucous membrane of the nose and sinuses secretes approximately two and one-half pints of mucus daily. Mucus may seem like a disgusting substance to most people, but they should understand that it plays a vital role in keeping the sinuses clean. The mucus is produced by secreting glands in the mucous membrane lining the nose and sinuses. Small beating hairs (cilia) on the mucous membrane sweep the mucus along, carrying with it all of the particulate matter, debris, bacteria, and so on, into the back of the nose. The mucus is then carried down the back of the throat, lubricating the mucous membrane, the throat, tongue, and larynx (voicebox). It also aids in the swallowing mechanism. When the nasal mucous membrane is irritated by either infectious or environmental conditions, the normal response of the nose and sinuses is to produce more mucus in an effort to dilute and wash away the offending irritating material. These irritating materials might be viral or bacterial infections, pollens, or other irritants in the environment.

The nose is a very reactive organ because it needs to respond by reflex to temperature changes and emotional states. The tissues of the nose are very richly supplied with blood vessels, and these may expand or contract in a moment's notice depending on the needs of the body. Upper respiratory infections and allergic responses are very common. Eighty percent of adults experience congestion, as well as decongestion, on a routine basis. Congestion and decongestion alternate from one side of the nose to the other. On average, the cycle lasts two and one-half hours, but cycles vary widely. This is a reflex mechanism controlled by the central nervous system. Since it is normal, most people are unaware of its occurrence.

Respiratory Infections

There are three common causes of nasal reactivity that produce nasal blockage and an increase in mucus production: viral upper respiratory infections, allergies, and vasomotor rhinitis, a condition caused by a variety of situations. Along with increased mucus production and blockage, a person may experience a sense of pressure or pain in or around the eyes and the forehead, or under the cheeks. This pressure is felt when two surfaces of mucous membranes press on one another in certain parts of the nasal cavity. This contact stimulates production of a chemical called "substance P," which produces pain in the nose or surrounding areas. The reactivity of the nasal mucous membrane can also produce headache in a susceptible individual. The headache is usually referred pain to the top of the head. However, the pain can be felt on the sides or back of the head as well.

Viral Infections

The most common causes of infection in both childhood and adulthood are viral upper respiratory infections. There are a number of viruses that can affect us, and they range in their degree of severity. These viruses can be spread in a variety of ways, by droplets, for example, such as in coughing or sneezing, or by direct contact. Even hugging, kissing, or touching an infected person can spread them. Some viruses can be spread by objects (a process doctors call *fomite transmission*). Infected individuals may touch objects, such as pencils, pens, silverware, dishes, or papers— just about anything; other people who pick up those objects and then rub their noses or eyes may transmit the virus or infectious element to themselves.

Viral infections in both adults and children progress by stages. In the initial, *irritating phase,* the nose itches and burns and produces lots of mucus material. In addition, the tissues in the nose might become swollen and cause nasal blockage. Virtually every one of us has experienced this during a common cold. The eyes tear and the ears feel stuffy. In two or three days, this irritative phase gives way to the *purulent phase,* in which the secretions can become yellow. The yellow color, indicating the death of cells within the nose, is also a valuable clue to doctors that there may be a secondary bacterial invasion. The purulent phase can last four to five days and should gradually clear in a normal individual. (This last phase is called the *resolution phase.*)

A simple respiratory infection caused by a virus can last from five to ten days, then clears spontaneously. But when bacteria cause the problem, it's altogether another story.

Bacterial Infections

In bacterial infections, the second, or purulent, phase usually is prolonged, and at this time one or more of the sinus cavities can become infected. Swollen mucous membranes prevent the secretions in the sinus from flowing out into the nose, and the mucus in the sinus becomes involved in an infection.

The initial treatment for a viral or bacterial infection is nasal decongestants, which can be taken as nasal sprays or by mouth. In addition, warm steam inhalations and the use of an acetaminophen product, such as Tylenol, in children or aspirin or aspirin-like medication in adults are helpful. If the sinus infection is not cleared with symptomatic management and if the sinus infection produces increasing pain, redness, swelling, and fever, an appropriate antibiotic has to be started. By this time you should have seen your physician. A worsening or prolongation of the problem should help determine the visit. Putting off the doctor visit will not accomplish anything in these cases because bacterial infections very rarely go away spontaneously. Oral antibiotic therapy is almost always necessary and is sufficient to cure a bacterial infection. During the seven-to-ten-day course of antibiotic therapy, the infection usually clears and the symptoms decrease.

Sinusitis

If a bacterial infection worsens and you are experiencing some of the problems given above, you may have *sinusitis*. Usually sinusitis can be complicated by a particularly severe infection or by an unusually vulnerable individual (an "immunocompromised person"). Diabetes or other systemic diseases, as well as HIV infection, can make a person vulnerable to an extension of the infection beyond the sinus cavities. Remember, the sinuses can interface with the brain, and infection sometimes spreads to the covering of the brain. *Meningitis,* an infection of the brain itself (called a brain abscess) can occur. Another possibility—although it is rare—is the infection of an eye socket. Although these conditions are not common, they offer additional reasons for seeing your doctor if sinus problems continue.

In some people, acute sinusitis may produce long-standing changes in the mucous membrane of the sinuses and of the sinus draining areas. These individuals' sinuses drain poorly and they become more susceptible to reinfection. Patients who have continuous and recurrent sinusitis may have underlying anatomic abnormalities, such as changes in the position of the nasal septum. Remember, the *nasal septum* usually lies in the middle of the nose; if it deviates from one side to the other, it produces changes in drainage patterns in the sinuses. In addition, allergies may make an individual more susceptible to the recurrent infections. Underlying anatomic and allergic diseases have to be ruled out in order to correct the recurring problems.

Acute sinusitis does not usually call for surgical intervention, but if it does not respond to antibiotic therapy and appears to be extending beyond the sinuses, then surgical drainage of them can be done. Before surgery is carried out, however, the patient's sinuses should be carefully examined by X rays and by CAT scan.

Surgeons can make surgical modifications of the sinus drainage sites by a variety of means. A new procedure is called *functional endoscopic sinus surgery* (FESS). This surgery can be carried out within the nose and does not require an external incision. Although FESS is not right for everyone, for individuals with specific sinus drainage problems, this technique provides an excellent means of interrupting the cycle of recurring sinus infections. Correction of a deviated nasal septum may also be required.

Allergies and Environmental Irritants

All of us have some form of allergy. In many cases it is barely noticed, but some individuals have an unusual capacity to respond to the materials in their environment—that is, some people will react to just about anything. These *atopic* individuals manifest the symptoms of an allergy. Genes determine that an individual is predisposed to allergies. Allergies may be of several types. One type is an *inhalant allergy*. The inhalant allergies are divided into two groups: seasonal allergens and allergens that persist year round. Seasonal allergies are related to the production of pollen and peoples' reactions to it. In early spring, tree pollens are the major allergen. In late spring, the allergen culprit is grasses, because they begin to pollinate at this time. During the summer months, many flowers and weeds pollinate, and all of them can cause an allergic response. In fall, ragweed sensitivity occurs, and in the winter months, when no pollination occurs, the most common persistent allergens are dust, dust mites, molds, and animal dander. If you are an allergic person, there is not a season that may not give you trouble.

The treatment of people for allergies, both adults and children, falls into three major categories: antihistamines, immunotherapy, and careful observation. Initially, if the allergies are minimal and sporadic, nothing needs to be done. If an individual has short bouts of allergies in spring or fall or is going to be exposed to an allergen for a relatively short time, however, antihistamines can manage or control the symptoms. Along with the antihistamine, medicated nasal sprays can be helpful in relieving nasal complaints.

Antihistamine

When a specific cell within the mucous membrane of the nose and sinuses reacts to a specific allergen, *histamine* is released. Histamine increases mucus production and produces swelling of the nasal mucous membrane tissues on the inside of the nose. These reactions can be blocked by *antihistamine*. Steroid nasal sprays, used with or without an antihistamine, also offer relief of the nasal symptoms. Antihistamines are generally very successful, but many individuals find that antihistamines make them sleepy or groggy and they cannot tolerate them. For these people physicians recommend allergy shots (*immunotherapy*). Immunotherapy can also be used by individuals whose allergies require taking large amounts of medication for a long time. Immunotherapy is different from antihistamines. The allergy shots are made up of a vaccine (*antigen*) that incorporates small amounts of the materials to which the peerson is sensitive (the *allergen*). In other words, a small amount of what causes an individual's allergic reaction is injected into his or her body; this stimulates the immune system to produce the substance that will block the allergic reaction. Immunotherapy is not simple, nor is it precise. Obviously, allergy shots cannot begin until the doctor can determine exactly what the individual is sensitive to.

Skin testing is the most precise way to determine what causes allergic reactions. In this technique, small amounts of a specific allergen are injected into the skin and the reaction (if any) is noted and recorded. Once the specific allergens that cause reactions are identified, a vaccine can be made and administered. About 85 percent of people with allergies can be helped by immunotherapy. It takes eight to twelve months of injection therapy, on a weekly or biweekly basis, in order to achieve good results.

Patients with allergies not only get symptoms of sneezing, runny nose, and nasal blockage but they also experience itching of the eyes and throat. Ear symptoms, with fullness, blockage, and fluid formation in the middle ear, can be another problem. In some people, the allergic response includes a reaction tht causes the mucous membrane to become thickened or to form little *polyps* (bits of tissue that are filled with fluid). Polyps can block the nasal passage by growing out of the sinuses and into the nasal cavity, decreasing airflow. At the same time, they can block sinus drainage, and poor drainage can cause the sinuses to become infected. If polyps do form and cause airway blockage and sinus drainage problems, they should be removed and the drainage portion of the sinuses should be opened.

Nonallergic Causes of Congestion

Another common cause of nasal congestion is a problem in the blood vessels, *vasomotor rhinitis*. *Vaso* refers to blood vessel, *motor* to forces, and *rhinitis* to the conditions of the nose. The abundant blood vessels of the nasal cavity, especially of the nasal airway, are under the control of the nervous system. Substances and conditions that affect the nervous system can thus affect nasal airway openness and mucus production. For example, medication for high blood pressure can cause nasal stuffiness. Sometimes another medication is substituted and the problem disappears. Although over-the-counter nasal spray can help relieve congestion temporarily, it can also make the problem worse if it is overused, causing a *rebound rhinitis,* which is increased congestion, perhaps leading to *profound nasal congestion.* For this reason, decongestant nasal drops and sprays should not be used for more than five consecutive days.

Hormones, such as estrogen, can affect blood vessel engorgement in the nose. Some women who take oral contraceptives complain of nasal congestion. When pregnancy raises natural estrogen levels, some women become quite disabled by congestion. Pregnant women who want to take *any* medication should check with their doctors first. Another hormonal cause of nasal congestion is *hypothyroidism,* a condition in which there is not enough thyroid hormone. These disorders should be treated in a manner that coordinates the efforts of the family doctor and an ear, nose, and throat specialist.

Life situations that produce such emotions an anxiety, hostility, guilt, or feelings of frustration and resentment also affect the nervous system and can disturb nasal blood flow balance. This type of nasal congestion and discharge may be chronic or intermittent. Nasal congestion may accompany a migraine headache; this explains why so many patients with migraine headaches are certain they have sinus headaches.

Some people report that exposure to irritating dust, gasses, propellants, and other air pollutants elicit a vasomotor reaction; the reaction might not be truly allergic, but nevertheless it creates nasal congestion. The most common of these irritants is tobacco smoke. The best treatment is avoidance or air filtration.

There are many causes of nasal congestion. All of us will suffer at some time from these problems, but it is important to realize that treatment is available and that one does not have to suffer for a prolonged period.

About the Author

Dr. Max Ronis is a professor and chair of the Department of Otolaryngology at the Temple University Health Sciences Center in Philadelphia. He received his medical degree from Temple University School of Medicine in 1956 and completed an internship and postgraduate training in otolaryngology at Temple

University Hospital. Dr. Ronis has maintained a clinical practice in Philadelphia since 1960.

He is a widely sought consultant in the treatment of disorders of the ears, nose, and throat and is a member of numerous general and otolaryngology medical societies on the local, regional, and national levels.

QUESTIONS FOR THE DOCTOR

Q: *My doctor told me that my child can't have a sinus infection in the first two years of life because the sinuses are not formed. When are the sinuses formed?*

A: Your doctor is partly correct. The maxillary and the ethmoid sinuses are both present in the newborn, but the maxillary sinuses do not become clinically significant until the child is eighteen to twenty-four months old. The frontal sinuses do not become present until the sixth year of life, and the sphenoid sinuses are not present until a child reaches age nine. Doctors are often concerned about sinus infections in young children. There is no reason to think that a young child might not be suffering from this problem.

Q: *How do I know I have a sinus infection?*

A: In an adult the most common symptoms of acute sinusitis are headache and facial pain. These symptoms may follow an upper respiratory infection. But facial pain and tenderness do not have to be present; in fact, sinus pain can masquerade as a toothache. That happens when the pain of the maxillary sinus is present. Maxillary sinus pain usually begins to occur within the first two hours after waking up, and by early afternoon it can become extremely painful. Usually maxillary sinus pain decreases as the evening approaches.

To examine someone with sinus tenderness, the doctor pushes on the areas surrounding the sinuses to see how tender they are. Next, he or she determines if the sinuses are full by means of a test called *transillumination*. In this test, light from a doctor's otoscope is used to see how empty (or full) the sinuses are. The degree of fullness often determines the approach to care. Sometimes it is not very easy to tell how full the sinuses are and the physician has to order X-ray studies of the sinuses. Transillumination is not a substitute for these X rays; it is a test that is far from perfect, but it is useful in deciding on the best treatment.

Q: *My doctor says my child has suffered from acute sinusitis. Is that the same problem we see in adults?*

A: Acute sinusitis in children is caused by many of the same bacteria that cause infections in adults. If a child has sinusitis, it is usually in the maxillary sinuses. Sinus infection in the frontal and sphenoid sinuses are quite rare. I mentioned that headache was one of the classic signs of acute sinusitis in adults, but headache and facial tenderness are extremely rare in children. Children with this infection usually have a persistent cough, fever, and runny nose. Doctors find it very difficult to tell if a child has a sinus infection and they may miss this infection in one out of three cases; however, the child usually does not suffer, because antibiotics are often given to treat associated infections and they serve a dual purpose by treating the sinus infection as well.

Q: *I have heard that antihistamines and decongestants can raise blood pressure. Is that true?*

A: Some of these medications *can* raise your blood pressure, so it is very important to ask your physician whether you should use them. People tend to think that because they can purchase medications over-the-counter, these medicines are safe. Just like prescribed medications, over-the-counter drugs are only safe if used with the knowledge of their side effects. There is nothing wrong with calling your doctor to see if he or she has any objection to your using over-the-counter medications. It is better for you to make sure the drug is safe than it is to risk a potential problem.

Q: *My child has asthma and seems to suffer from sinusitis as well. Is there a connection between the two?*

A: As physicians learn more about sinusitis, we are realizing that there may be a relationship between asthma and sinusitis. In fact, in one recent study of patients with both sinusitis and asthma, more than 90 percent had sinusitis that occurred before the asthma attack. More research needs to be done in this area.

Q: *Why do we get sinus infections?*

A: There are four common causes of sinusitis. In the classic case, sinusitis follows viral infections, in particular, upper respiratory infections. That is because the sinus openings can be blocked by inflammation and swelling caused by the infection. Allergy and nasal polyps can also lead to blockages. Another cause of sinusitis is the accumulation of mucus or fluid in the sinuses. Remember, bacteria flourish in warm, moist places, and sinus fluid provides a great medium for bacterial growth. Sometimes the bacteria begin to grow in the sinus fluid and the swelling continues, and before you know it, there is a buildup of pressure in the sinuses. A third cause of sinusitis is viral damage to the respiratory cilia, the hairs that help move debris in and out of the sinus region; when they are damaged, mucus and bacteria might not be cleared out properly. A final cause is dental infections.

Q: *What bacteria are usually found in sinus infections?*
A: Two common bacteria, *streptococcus pneumoniae* and *hemophilus influenzae,* are often found in sinus infections. Many antibiotics are very effective for treating these.

Q: *How do you tell whether someone has a simple headache or a headache caused by a sinus infection?*
A: It is difficult to tell when one is having a sinus headache because some headaches have symptoms that include pressure and pain in the region of the sinuses. The key to determining which kind is to find out the history of the headache. Often the most important clues are where and when the pain occurs.

Q: *Why are X rays obtained in cases of suspected sinusitis?*
A: The real advantage of X rays is that they can allow doctors to see fluid levels in the sinuses. A series of X rays showing the head in different positions is usually necessary. X rays can also be very valuable because they can help physicians tell if their treatment is curing the sinusitis. X rays often indicate that the sinuses need to be drained. CAT scans can also add to the X ray information, but these are generally used only for the most serious cases.

Q: *My doctor told me to take my medication lying down in bed. I couldn't understand why I had to do this.*
A: Doctors often tell their patients that to apply nose drops they should lie on their backs with their heads hanging over the edge of a bed. They turn to one side and apply nose drops to that side of the nose, then do the same thing for the other side. This method allows the medication to penetrate into the upper parts of the nasal cavities and the other areas of the sinuses. The medication in nose drops is usually a *vasoconstrictor,* which reduces swelling of the blood vessels. This method of application can improve the effectiveness of the decongestants and promote drainage. Remember, you should use these types of nose drops (or nasal sprays) for only three or four days; after longer use there may be a rebound phenomenon, with increased congestion after the drugs wear off.

Inhalation of hot water vapor (steam) can help loosen nasal mucus and relieve the symptoms of nasal congestion. You can get excellent results by using very hot water from your shower or bath to fill the room with steam. A more energy-saving approach is to fill a large bowl with hot water, drape your head and the bowl with a towel, and breathe in the steam. Of course, you should be careful about coming into contact with steam, because it can cause severe burns.

Q: I saw two doctors. The first said my child had otitis media, an ear infection and the second said my child didn't. How could one have a different opinion than the other?

A: There are several problems in examining a child with an ear infection. Doctors generally begin by using an otoscope to look into the ear. It is difficult to see whether there is an ear infection, even though this instrument is used. We usually look for a reddening of the eardrum (a structure inside the ear canal that looks like a drum) or for swelling or pressure behind that area. Earwax or a child's movement can make it difficult for physicians to get a good look. Even when things are perfectly visible, the degree of rednes might be interpreted differently by two doctors. Some physicians begin to treat the infection immediately, even in uncertain situations, rather than to wait for the symptoms to worsen. Others wait, preferring not to medicate the patient until they are sure infection is present.

Parents can follow a few basic guidelines to tell whether the child might have an ear infection. The following are some signs to look for in a child: Notice whether the child pulls on one or both ears (ear infections can be quite painful; and if the child has been pulling on his or her ears or has been crying, he or she might be in pain). Many patients with an acute ear infection do not have ear pain, however, so patients and doctors have to be careful to not use pain as the only criteria. An elevated temperature is often a symptom of an ear infection, so check the child's temperature.

Q: My child seems to have an ear infection every month. Should something be done, besides administering antibiotics every time there is an infection?

A: This is a very delicate situation because different physicians often handle the problem differently. If your child is suffering from several ear infections a year, you may need to consider other measures of treatment. One measure includes the use of *chronic antibiotic therapy* to suppress bacteria. A child takes a reduced dose of a medication known to fight ear infections over a long period of time. The hope is that the bacteria can be suppressed from growing and causing the infection. Another option is to put tubes into your child's eardrums.

This procedure helps reduce the fluid and pressure behind the drums, which can be a cause of difficulty.

Q: *My doctor told me not to have my child drink his bottle lying on his back. Why?*

A: When your child swallows, he or she may affect the pressure in the region of the middle ear. This pressure change can cause secretions to go where they shouldn't; thus you should always elevate the head of a child when he or she is drinking.

Q: *Why is it so important for my child to be treated for ear infections?*

A: Chronic ear infections can cause problems with both speech and hearing. (It is critical to have your child evaluated for these problems.) Another reason to be concerned about ear infections in children is the possibility that an infection can spread to other parts of the body. Meningitis, mentioned previously, is also a concern. Your pediatrician or family physician needs to know when your child has a serious problem. Your child's health can be protected by quick intervention. In many cases, the only way to effect a cure is to treat the problem right away.

Q: *When is a sore throat a problem?*

A: A sore throat becomes a problem when it hurts and causes difficulty swallowing or speaking. It may be caused by irritation from postnasal drip during allergy season or from cigarette smoking. A bacterial cause can be the first warning that a serious infection is on the way, however. Doctors often have to determine whether a bacterial infection or a virus is causing the sore throat. If such symptoms as a cough, runny nose, and hoarseness are present along with the sore throat, something other than a bacterial infection may be the cause. If someone has a sore throat but does not have any of the other symptoms, a bacteria such as *streptococcus* (strep) may be the cause. A careful examination is important. The doctor may order a throat culture to determine the cause of the sore throat. Strep infection is one possible cause of a sore throat (strep throat). It is most common in children between age five and fifteen; it is very rare in those people under age three and over age thirty. Strep cases are usually limited to winter and spring. Strep throat should be strongly suspected whenever the patient has a temperature greater than 101 degrees or has swollen glands.

Q: *My doctor says that I am a chronic carrier of strep. Is this bad for me?*

A: Well, you are not alone. About 15 percent of the population carries the streptococcus bacteria on a chronic basis. When your doctor tests you for any sort of throat infection, the odds are that the test will be positive for strep. Because of this, you may be put on antibiotics on a consistent basis every time you have a complaint. Physicians suspect that a person is a chronic carrier of streptococcus if he or she always seems to have positive tests.

Q: *Is strep infection the only bacteria that can cause throat problems?*
A: No, in fact physicians consider other causes of infection, including gonorrhea, in patients who are sexually active with more than one partner. In some undergraduate populations, gonorrhea is almost as common as strep throat as a cause of sore throat. Thus the symptoms of the immediate problem (the sore throat) might be less serious than is the potential for other problems; many doctors use such situations as an opportunity to stress important public health points. For example, a doctor discussing the possible causes of a sore throat to people who are sexually active may emphasize the risks of HIV infection and other sexually transmitted diseases.

14

Skin Conditions and Disorders

Scott M. Panzer, M.D.

Dermatology involves the diagnosis and treatment of diseases and conditions of the skin, hair, and nails, which together form the single largest organ system of the human body. The three layers of this complex organ are the epidermis, dermis, and subcutaneous tissue. The *epidermis,* the outer layer of the skin visible to the eye, is itself composed of several cell types; the most plentiful are *keratinocytes,* and the ones that give skin its pigmentation or color are *melanocytes.* The *dermis,* the middle layer, gives skin much of its strength and elasticity (the ability to bounce back like a rubber band when stretched). The dermis is made up of collagen and elastic fibers, as well as blood vessels (for nourishment and heat regulation), nerves (for sensation of touch, pressure, temperature, itching, and pain), sweat and sebaceous (oil-producing) glands, hair follicles (which produce hair), and various cells that migrate to the skin from the blood. The *subcutaneous tissue,* or fatty layer, is the deepest part of the skin. Although many of us are concerned about keeping this layer to a minimum (and exercise to do so), we should be aware that it does serve a useful purpose, as a source of energy when our reserves are low and as insulation against heat loss. When any of these components of the skin change and become abnormal, the skin condition or disease requires treatment.

Because the skin is the largest and most visible of our organs, it is not surprising that *dermatology* largely involves the observation and description of the problem, which frequently is sufficient to make a diagnosis.

Dermatologists have developed a descriptive language to evaluate skin changes, which makes the diagnostic process more objective and uniform. The basic lesions, or abnormal changes in the skin's structure, are known as *primary lesions*. Read through the definitions of the following terms to get a sense of the range of lesions and refer back to the list as you read about the specific diseases in the remainder of the chapter.

macule: a flat discoloration of the skin; for example, a freckle

papule: a raised solid lesion up to 1cm in diameter; for example, a raised mole

plaque: a raised, superficial, solid lesion more than 1cm in diameter; for example, a lesion caused by psoriasis

nodule: a raised solid lesion, with the deeper dermal portion more than 1cm in diameter; for example, a lipoma (a benign fatty growth)

vesicle: a collection of free fluid up to 1cm in diameter (a small blister); for example, a blister from herpes simplex (a cold sore on the lips)

bulla: a collection of free fluid more than 1cm in diameter (a large blister); for example, a large blister from bullous impetigo (a bacterial infection of the skin)

pustule: a collection of white blood cells and free fluid (commonly known as pus); for example, a pimple caused by acne

There are hundreds of skin conditions currently known to exist. I have selected five of the most common and will discuss why they occur, their pathogenesis (their origin and development), how to prevent (if possible) or minimize the problem, and how to treat the condition— either with over-the-counter products or with prescription medication or surgery under the care of your dermatologist, primary care physician, or surgeon.

Acne

Acne is a skin condition that commonly affects males and females, beginning in adolescence. It is often dismissed by parents as a minor affliction or as a normal part of the growing process and thus is not deemed worthy of treatment. This lack of timely treatment can lead to permanent scarring of the skin and to psychological damage. The unsightliness of both the active acne and its resultant "ice pick" type indented and papular or nodular (raised) scars causes many people embarrassment, lack of self-esteem, and depression. Scarring and psychological harm can both be avoided by treatment.

Acne can affect the face, chest, and back, because hair follicles in these locations contain the largest and most numerous oil-producing (sebaceous) glands. Acne is considered a multifactorial condition; that is, several different abnormalities occurring together cause the acne lesions to appear. The first lesions to appear are "whiteheads" and "blackheads," known collectively as *comedones,* which occur because a collection of oil, bacteria, and dead epidermal skin cells (keratinocytes) clog the pores. Although whiteheads and blackheads can develop at any time in life, they are particularly common at puberty because the sex hormone testosterone and its active metabolite dihydrotestosterone (DHT) increase the production of oil in the skin. This plugging of the pores allows specific bacteria (*P. acnes*) to grow deep in the hair follicle. Using the oil as its food supply, the bacteria proliferate, eventually causing rupture of the hair follicle. This rupture causes a collection of white blood cells to travel from the blood to this site, and the resultant inflammation produces the red nodules, papules, and yellow pustules commonly seen in acne.

Acne attacks some people more than others. It appears that the development of acne is mostly an inherited tendency and not particularly related to diet or to poor hygiene, as is commonly believed. Acne generally worsens during times of stress. For some women, it worsens before a menstrual period, perhaps because of a change in hormone levels. In rare instances, certain medications can make acne worse.

There are several effective treatments for acne. For mild conditions, it can be helpful to wash with soap and water to remove surface oil and to use over-the-counter products containing benzoyl peroxide, salicylic acid, or sulphur. For mild-to-moderate acne, prescription medications including topically applied antibiotics (erythromycin or clindamycin), retinoic acid (known as Retin-A), and benzoyl peroxide preparations are usually very helpful. For moderate-to-severe acne, which is often associated with some scarring, physicians may prescribe oral antibiotics such as tetracycline, erythromycin, doxycycline, minocycline, and others. If other drugs fail, some patients with severe, difficult-to-control acne can be treated with a course of Accutane, but this medication needs to be used only under the watchful eye of an experienced dermatologist because of its potential side effects. Fertile women, for example, must not be pregnant and pregnancy must be prevented while taking Accutane because of a very high risk of birth defects. Future treatment may consist of hormonal manipulation to block either the production or the action of acne-inducing hormones (such as DHT, mentioned previously).

Warts

Warts are skin-colored, tan, or red papules and plaques found on the skin and mucous membranes that are caused by a virus known as the human papilloma virus (HPV). Most people are infected with HPV at some time during their lives, and warts are particularly common in childhood. Sites of minor trauma, such as hands and feet, are frequently involved. Warts are often named by their location: *Plantar warts* occur on the soles, but *genital warts* (also known as *condylomata acuminata*) occur on and around the vagina or the penis, as well as on the nearby anus and surrounding skin. Other warts are named by their shape: *Flat warts* are barely felt with light touch, but *filiform* warts are long and pointy.

HPV infects the epidermis of the skin, but only in humans. The fact that other animals are not affected has made it difficult to study the infectivity of HPV. For example, warts can be transmitted by human's skin-to-skin contact, but it is unclear just how long the virus can survive when it is no longer on its human host (such as when it is on the floor of a locker room or on the deck of a swimming pool). Though many people with warts note that they have a relative or friend with warts who may have been the source, most individuals are unaware of where they picked up the HPV. Still, it makes sense to avoid direct skin contact, if possible, with anyone else's warts.

Genital warts differ from other warts mainly in the way that they are transmitted from one person to another. Most commonly, genital warts are found in adult men and women. They are usually, but not always, sexually transmitted. In other words, the virus is passed from one partner to the other during sexual intercourse, when the skin and mucous membranes (moist body cavities such as the vagina, anus, and mouth) come in contact. Small breaks in the skin, often microscopic, caused by the friction of the sex act make the chance of transmission quite high. In one study, about 50 percent of the male partners of women with genital warts were found to have genital warts as well, although most of the men were unaware of this because the warts were quite small. The risk of transmission of the HPV from one partner to another can be reduced by use of a condom, provided that it does not break and that it remains in place as a barrier between the skin of the infected and noninfected partner.

Genital warts should *not* be ignored. Whereas most warts are benign growths that are treatable and that will often go away even without treatment (particularly those in children), HPV has been strongly associated with cervical cancer in women. Though most women with genital warts will never develop cancer of the cervix, exposure to certain HPV types may place a woman at greater risk. Although HPV can be typed in a research lab (more than sixty types, designated type 1, type 2, etc., are already known), HPV typing is not generally available. Moreover, science has not yet determined the true risk of cervical cancer of a specific HPV type. So until the risk factors are clearly understood, most experts recommend that women with a history of genital warts be screened for cervical cancer by having a pelvic exam and a Pap smear at six-month to twelve-month intervals. In certain cases, colposcopy, the microscopic examination of the cervix usually performed by a gynecologist, can find evidence of HPV infection even when the Pap smear is normal or only mildly abnormal.

Recent studies of different forms of skin cancer have found evidence of HPV in some basal cell and squamous cell skin cancers (these cancers are discussed in detail in a later section of this chapter). These studies have not yet determined how common HPV is in these types of skin cancers; the cancers are largely thought to be caused by chronic sun exposure, and it is possible that the virus and the sun together induce some of them. A similar situation is seen in individuals with a rare inherited skin condition (known as *epidermodysplasia verruciformis*) in which hundreds of warts may cover the skin, and, not uncommonly, some of these warts turn into squamous cell skin cancer.

Numerous methods are used to deal with warts, depending on the site of the wart, the response to prior treatments, the numbers of warts, and the age of the patient, among other factors. Initial therapy often consists of salicylic acid (over-the-counter or prescription-strength) used daily for weeks to months. It is inexpensive and fairly painless. Other treatments include acids applied by a physician (bichloracetic or trichloracetic salicylic or pyruvic acid), destruction by freezing with liquid nitrogen, injection into the wart with the anticancer drug bleomycin, immunotherapy with a substance that causes a localized allergic reaction, indirectly destroying the wart (DNCB or SADE), occlusive treatment with waterproof tape, or surgical treatment by scraping and burning (curettage and electrodesiccation), excision, or laser destruction. Nevertheless, some warts recur no matter what physicians do. Unfortunately, it is impossible to know in advance whether one is dealing with an easily cured wart or one that is going to be resistant to therapy. With patience on the part of both patient and doctor, however, most warts will eventually go away on their own.

Psoriasis

Psoriasis is a chronic skin condition that affects approximately 3 percent of the population. The lesions of psoriasis are red papules and plaques, with a thick white scale or flaking on the surface. Although it can occur anywhere on the skin, body sites most often involved are the elbows, knees, and scalp. Occasionally, in questionable cases, the presence of small pits or indentations in the fingernails or toenails can help to determine the diagnosis. Itching is variable, from minimal to severe. Psoriasis may begin in infancy or it may appear at adolescence or at any time in one's adult life. Fifty percent of those with psoriasis have at least one other family member with the same condition; therefore, inheritance is believed to play a part in an individual's risk of developing it. Certain infections may worsen or may be associated with the onset of psoriasis. The most closely linked is "strep" infection, usually a cold or upper respiratory tract infection due to the organism *streptococcus pyogenes*. Other infections, such as candida, a type of yeast, may also cause psoriasis to worsen, especially in the skin folds (such as those in the armpits, under the breasts, or in the groin).

Dermatologists are not sure what causes psoriasis, but research is currently in progress to test the value of current theories to explain its development and severity. As noted above, infections may stimulate the immune system by releasing substances called antigens, which may leave the blood stream and become deposited in the skin. This, in turn, may be the stimulus for the inflammation and rapid epidermal cell division seen with psoriasis. It was thought for many years that psoriasis was primarily an abnormality of the epidermal skin cells, which mature and divide very quickly in psoriatic skin compared to normal skin. Recently, rapid clearing of psoriasis with cyclosporin, a drug that blocks the immune system (an immunomodulator) has led researchers to consider psoriasis as an abnormal immune response in the skin, with the rapid cell growth and division perhaps a secondary phenomenon. Drugs such as lithium and the beta-blocker class of blood pressure medication, as well as excess alcohol intake, can cause a flare-up of psoriasis in predisposed people. Also, stress can worsen psoriasis in some individuals.

Although there is no known cure for psoriasis, many effective treatments exist. For localized mild psoriasis, such as with elbow and knee involvement, topical cortisone creams and ointments of various strengths can be used for control, as well as injections of cortisone into small but resistant areas. A preparation known as anthralin (Drithocreme) applied on the psoriasis patches is a nonsteroidal alternative. Moisturizers, creams that contain salicylic acid, and topical tar products are also of some benefit.

For those with extensive skin involvement—between 15 percent and 100 percent of the skin surface—more aggressive treatment to clear the psoriasis is required. Several choices exist. For example, phototherapy in a dermatologist's office using ultraviolet B light (UVB phototherapy) or an oral medication combined with ultraviolet A light (PUVA photochemotherapy) would be effective for treating large areas of involved skin. Two powerful oral medications include methotrexate and etretinate, which are either taken alone or in combination with other therapies. Any of these treatments may cause significant side effects, and you should discuss with your physician the risks versus the benefits of treatment; only after this discussion can appropriate and individualized therapy be started.

Atopic Dermatitis

Atopic dermatitis (AD), commonly known as "eczema" is a disease that causes itchy, flaking, pink-to-red skin. It usually begins in childhood, often in infancy, with dry, itchy, scaly skin, especially involving the inner elbows and backs of the knees, the neck, and the face. In severe cases, most of the skin surface may be involved. Between 3 percent and 10 percent of the population has at least mild symptoms of AD. This condition is often chronic in childhood, but most children outgrow AD by early adult life. Unfortunately, for those more severely affected, this condition may persist well into the adult years.

People with AD often have family members with AD or a personal or family history of asthma or hay fever. For this reason, it is felt that AD, asthma, and hay fever are related inherited conditions. People with AD may have worsening symptoms with certain environmental exposures, for example, with irritating substances such as soaps and perfumes, low or extremely high humidity, skin infections, heat, sweating, and emotional stress. A specific food is rarely a source of flare-ups, but this can be investigated by an allergist if it is strongly suspected.

Generally, people with AD can minimize symptoms by avoiding harsh soaps, bathing with warm (not hot) water, and by using a cream- or ointment-based moisturizer immediately after gently toweling dry. To isolate specific triggers of symptoms, you can first eliminate any suspected skin irritants and then retry them one at a time on a small area of skin to see if the substance causes more itching or an inflamed rash. If a flare-up occurs, this product should be avoided.

In the winter months, a humidifier in the bedroom will help prevent the excessive skin dryness that results from the dry heat found in most homes. It is best to wear cotton clothing; synthetic fabrics, such as polyester, should be worn with caution and should be set aside if they appear to increase itching. Wool clothing is very irritating and should be avoided.

Many people with mild AD can control their condition most of the time by following these suggestions. At times of flare-up, however, regardless of the cause, stronger medicines are often needed. Cortisone (steroid) creams and ointments help stop the inflammation that leads to itching and are effective at times of flare-up. They vary widely in strength and should be used only as directed by a physician. For example, milder cortisone is needed for the face and skin folds (such as elbows, armpits, neck, and groin) and a stronger-than-average cortisone may be needed for other sites, such as the hands and feet. Use of stronger cortisone creams on the face and skin folds may lead to thinning of the skin (known as atrophy), with a wrinkled or shiny appearance of the skin and increased small surface blood vessels as well as an acne-like rash on the face. Excessive use of strong topical cortisone products over large body areas for more than a few weeks can be dangerous because they may suppress your body's own normal daily cortisone production by the adrenal glands.

Antihistamines taken by mouth, such as the prescription medicine hydroxyzine (Vistaril, Atarax) and the over-the-counter medication diphenhydramine (Benadryl), can help control itching temporarily but in many cases they may cause drowsiness. Antihistamines can be very helpful in preventing nighttime scratching and the insomnia that is associated with the itching. The dosage and frequency should be discussed with your doctor.

Skin infections, such as *folliculitis* (pustules of the hair follicles), boils, and *impetigo*, with honey-colored crusting, may either cause a flare-up of AD or may be the result of AD. Usually the organism, *staphylococcus aureus* (commonly called staph infection) is responsible for this. Antibiotics, such as erythromycin and dicloxacillin, are helpful in clearing the infection as well as in improving the itching and rash.

For severe flare-ups of AD, cortisone in a pill or injection form may be needed to break the cycle of itching, scratching, and inflammation. Although cortisone is very effective, long-term use has many possible side effects. Physicians thus advise short-term courses, and only when they are truly needed. Finally, light therapy, either with UVB or PUVA, as mentioned under psoriasis therapy, is at times quite helpful for those with severe atopic dermatitis.

Skin Cancer

The three main types of skin cancer, basal cell carcinoma, squamous cell carcinoma, and malignant melanoma, differ in the type of cell they arise from, the sites they commonly affect, the proper treatment, and the associated morbidity and mortality they cause.

Basal Cell Carcinoma

Basal cell carcinoma (BCC) is the most common skin cancer; in fact, it is the most commonly occurring cancer type. About 98 percent of BCCs are found on sun-exposed skin, especially that of the face, shoulders, upper chest, back and forearms, and legs. Risk factors for BCC include a family history of BCC and excessive sun exposures, especially in those who burn easily and tan poorly and have blue eyes and light-colored hair. BCC is named for the cell type that composes the tumor. Basal cells are the bottom-most layer of the epidermis. In BCC these cells grow in an uncontrolled way and invade the dermis (middle skin layer) and, eventually, the deeper tissues.

Suspect BCC when you have nonhealing sores that are present for more than a few weeks, lesions that bleed spontaneously or with minor injury, or scabs that come and go in the same location. Also be suspicious and consult a doctor if you find red-to-pearl-colored papules, white scar-like areas that arise without known cause, or flat, slowly enlarging, red scaly patches that vary in size from the barely visible to the size of a grapefruit.

The one risk factor of BCC that you can control is your degree of sun exposure. It has been said that most people experience more than 50 percent of their lifetime sun exposure by age eighteen. This shows that the people who may benefit most from sun protection are children who have not already had the bulk of their lifetime exposure.

Certainly, many adults today can rightfully say that they were not advised to protect against excessive sun exposure while growing up because, until relatively recently, little was known about the damaging cumulative effects of the sun's ultraviolet light. Today's children and teenagers cannot make that claim, and yet many ignore the warnings and continue to sunbathe to achieve an "attractive" tan. For those who feel the need to look tan, artificial tanning creams and lotions with the active ingredient dihydroxyacetone can safely give the look of a tan without the sun damage caused by traditional tanning.

You can avoid excessive sun exposure in many ways. When possible, planning outdoor activities before 10 a.m. or after 2 p.m. will avoid exposure during the periods of greatest ultraviolet light intensity. Shading oneself with a hat during outside activities such as gardening or golfing or under an umbrella while at the beach or by wearing a t-shirt after swimming are good practices that should become habits. The routine use of sunscreens on exposed skin is also advisable, particularly on spring and summer days when more than thirty minutes of outdoor activities are planned, and even on cloudy days, because ultraviolet light can penetrate clouds even when visible light is blocked. (More information about sunscreens follows in "Questions for the Doctor.")

Therapy for BCCs usually calls for one of several surgical methods, performed after numbing the skin with local anesthetic. Most commonly, surgeons use a technique of scraping away the tumor with a sharp instrument, followed by burning of the base (known by the medical term *electrodesiccation and curettage*). Deep excision, that is, cutting away the tumor, followed by stitching the wound closed is also commonly performed. Both methods have an overall comparable cure rate of greater than 95 percent on BCCs that have not been previously treated. Physicians use laser treatment and liquid nitrogen freezing less frequently, but they are also effective ways of destroying the tumor. *Mohs microscopically controlled surgery*, performed by specially trained dermatologic surgeons, produces the highest cure rate, but expense and time factors make this treatment most suitable for recurrent skin cancers and large skin cancers.

Finally, radiation therapy can be curative for those individuals with BCC who are not good surgical candidates.

People with a history of BCC should have their skin examined at least once or twice a year once their surgical scar has healed. This is to check for a return of the skin cancer at the surgery site as well as to search for any new skin cancers. This monitoring enables physicians to begin treatment when the tumor is small, which, in turn, means an easier cure and less scarring. Though BCCs rarely spread through the bloodstream to distant sites (metastasize), if left untreated, they can destroy the skin and any surrounding structures, including the eyes and nose.

Squamous Cell Carcinoma

Squamous cell carcinoma (SCC), the second most common form of skin cancer, occurs about one-sixth as often as BCC. It appears primarily on sun-exposed sites, as does BCC; in addition to the sites of involvement previously mentioned in connection with BCC, it occurs on the lower lip, the inside of the mouth (particularly in tobacco users), and at sites of scars (both surgical and traumatic). SCC may occur many years after exposure to other carcinogens, such as radiation therapy (using X rays for treatment of a prior tumor or condition) or arsenic ingestion (used many years ago for various ailments).

SCC is named from its abnormally growing cell type, the squamous cell, which normally makes up the bulk of the epidermis, or outer layer of the skin. In SCC a change occurs in which unlimited growth causes invasion of first the dermis and later the deeper tissues. Sometimes the tumor will be spread by the bloodstream to distant sites. Known as *metastatic SCC,* this is potentially life-threatening at this stage.

Squamous cell carcinoma often appears as papules or nodules (bumps of varying sizes), which may be scabbed or warty on the surface and may bleed spontaneously or with minor trauma. SCC may also appear as flat, nonhealing areas, with the skin scaly and red, eroded, or ulcerated. Since early treatment is usually curative and late treatment poses the risk of metastases, any suspicious lesion should be examined sooner rather than later by your dermatologist or primary doctor.

Since the vast majority of SCCs are sun-induced, if you follow the advice mentioned above about the prevention of BCC, you can help prevent this form of skin cancer as well. SCCs are treated in the same fashion as are BCCs.

Malignant Melanoma

Malignant melanoma (MM) is the least-common but most-serious form of skin cancer because of its tendency to metastasize. If it does metastasize, it is often incurable and fatal. By the year 2000 it is estimated that one in one hundred fair-skinned individuals will develop MM during their lifetimes. When MM is diagnosed early and completely removed, it is curable in well over 90 percent of cases.

MM is named for the cell type that forms the tumor, the *melanocyte.* This cell type is evenly distributed throughout the skin and is also present in benign collections, commonly called moles. MM is a result of a cancerous change in one or more melanocytes, which leads to unrestricted growth of these cells. Although initially confined to the epidermis, these uncontrolled cells eventually spread to the dermis. Blood vessels in the dermis may then transport the MM cells to distant sites, a process known as *metastatic melanoma.* Since no treatment of this late stage of melanoma has proven effective, the goal must be for early detection and removal of these cancers.

MMs may arise from previously normal-appearing moles that become cancerous or may appear on otherwise normal-appearing skin without a preexisting mole. The changes to look for in MM are as easy to remember as ABCD.

> **A** stands for asymmetry; that is, a mole growing in only one portion is suspect. It might become more raised focally or may spread out on the skin surface at one edge. In contrast, normal moles are round or oval and are not significantly more raised in one portion than another.

> **B** is for border. MMs often have a fuzzy, irregular, or scalloped border; ordinary moles have a distinct border between the mole and the surrounding skin.

> **C** is for color. Two or more shades of brown or additional colors of red, black, or white are often present in MMs. Ordinary moles are fairly uniform in color throughout.

> **D** is for diameter. Most ordinary moles that occur after the first few months of life are less than six millimeters in diameter, which is roughly the size of a pencil eraser. MMs are usually, but not always, larger than six millimeters.

Risk factors for MM development include: a fair complexion that easily burns, that poorly tans, and that freckles with sun exposure; blue eyes and blond or red hair; the presence of many normal-appearing moles; the presence of several atypical moles (moles that share some of the features of MM but are benign); or a family history of melanoma. MM occurs more commonly on sun-exposed skin (back, face, and legs more often in women) than sun-protected sites (buttocks or breasts). However, MM can occur anywhere on the skin surface, including the mucous membranes (inside the mouth). Therefore, though sun exposure plays a role in the development of MM, it is not the only factor. It has also been proposed that one or a few severe burns, often in childhood, may be as important as the cumulative lifetime sun exposure as a risk factor for MM. Despite our incomplete knowledge, we can say that avoidance of excess sun exposure probably reduces the risk of MM and certainly reduces the risk of both BCC and SCC. It cannot be emphasized enough that *early detection and removal of skin cancer*, especially MM, *can save lives.*

The five most common skin problems can all be treated successfully, provided that treatment begins early. Even those conditions that are not life-threatening may have long-term consequences that are best avoided.

About the Author

Dr. Scott M. Panzer attended Franklin and Marshall College and the University of Pennsylvania. He received his medical degree from Temple University. Dr. Panzer completed his dermatology residency at the University of North Carolina–Chapel Hill and is Diplomate of the American Board of Dermatology and a fellow of the American Academy of Dermatology.

He is currently president of the Delaware Academy of Dermatology and is in private practice in Newark, Delaware.

QUESTIONS FOR THE DOCTOR

Q: *What strength of sunscreen (SPF) should I use?*
A: Sunscreens are ranked by their sun protection factor (SPF), currently ranging from 2 to 50. The higher the number, the greater the degree of protection against the sun's harmful ultraviolet B (UVB) rays. An SPF 15 sunscreen will block 14/15 or 93 percent of the UVB light, which is sufficient for most people. Those who burn in spite of adequate application of an SPF 15 sunscreen (which includes reapplication if swimming or perspiring heavily) or who have a sun-sensitive

condition such as lupus, might choose a higher SPF sunscreen for even greater protection. For most people, the higher rating (and higher cost) is not needed. The key to sunscreen protection is coating all of the areas exposed, such as the face, ears, neck, forearms, tops of the hands, and so forth, and reapplying the sunscreen as needed.

Q: *How often should I reapply my sunscreen?*
A: That depends on your activities and the sunscreen used. Sunscreens marked as waterproof should stay in place for eighty minutes of immersion in water; those marked water-resistant are protective for forty minutes of water immersion. Sweat-resistant sunscreens provide protection for thirty minutes of heavy perspiration. After these time intervals, it is best to reapply the sunscreen for maximum protection. Other sunscreens not specifically marked as waterproof, water-resistant, or sweat-resistant may wash off quickly after a short swim and, if you do not reapply them, a false sense of security may cause you to overexpose yourself and develop an unwanted sunburn.

Q: *Is ultraviolet A [UVA] light, found in the equipment in tanning salons, safer than UVB?*
A: The more we learn about UVA light, the more we realize the damage it can cause. In natural sunlight, UVA is much more plentiful than UVB. It is this type of ray that causes most of a suntan, and it is the only light source allowed for tanning salons. UVA light penetrates the skin more deeply than does UVB light, and animals exposed to UVA and UVB are more likely to develop skin tumors than those receiving UVB alone. This means that UVA and UVB light are synergistic, or more than just additive, in their ability to promote cancers in animals. The above suggests that UVA exposure, either from tanning salons or from natural sunlight, adds to your overall risk of skin cancer.

This suggestion of added risk has led sunscreen manufacturers to pay attention increasingly to UVA protection, and several brands list protection against UVA on their labels. Currently, the question of how to reproducibly measure a sunscreen's UVA protection is being worked out so that sun protection factors can be standardized for UVA in the same way as they are for UVB. The most effective UVA protecting sunscreen on the market today is sold with the brand name Photoplex. It blocks more than 90 percent of the sun's UVA rays and also carries an SPF rating of 15 against UVB rays. It is available in pharmacies without a prescription, but you might have to ask for it by name. Among those that can benefit most from this product are people with a specific sun sensitivity that may be in the UVA spectrum, such as those with lupus or melasma (commonly known as the "mask of pregnancy").

Q: *I recently read a report that sunscreens are unsafe and can actually increase the risk of skin cancer. Is this true?*

A: Sunscreens can only help prevent skin cancer by blocking the sun's dangerous rays. The study was saying that many people use these creams inappropriately. They stay in the sun for extended periods of time or do not reapply them. Other methods of preventing sun exposure, such as wearing a wide-brim hat, long-sleeved shirt, and long pants, may be as effective at preventing the overexposure. In other words, use common sense. Sunscreens are an aid; they are not a cure-all. Clearly, it is advantageous to use sunscreen with an SPF of 15 or greater.

Q: *It is safe for me to take my baby to the beach in the summer?*

A: Yes, but a qualified yes. You may bring your baby to the beach for a short period of time, but you should keep your baby shielded from the sun. No matter how dark your skin is, your baby's skin is extremely sensitive to the sun, and it should be protected. You should speak with your pediatrician to ask if he or she suggests using a sun block for your child. There are other problems in addition to sunburn associated with sun exposure. For example, because of the heat, a child can become dehydrated quite rapidly, and you need to continually replenish his or her fluid. If you are going to take your child to the beach or to any sunny area, you have to be extremely sensitive about your child's needs.

Q: *Can I get sunburned when I am swimming in the ocean?*

A: Yes! In fact, you are probably more at risk than if you were just on the beach. This is because you feel the sun's direct rays as well as the reflections of those rays. Many of the most severe sunburns are the result of people thinking they are safe from sunburn when they are in the water.

Q: *My doctor told me I have scabies and gave me a cream to use to treat it. I've used the cream and the condition doesn't seem to be getting any better. Could he have made the wrong diagnosis?*

A: Possibly the treatment did not treat the scabies effectively the first time around. In many cases physicians have to treat a disease two or three times before we cure it. *Scabies* is caused by a parasitic mite (*Sarcoptes scabiei*) infestation. The infestation causes people to itch, seeming much worse at night. Usually scabies affects the genitalia, lower abdomen, or the wrists and the finger webs, but it can occur in other places such as the legs, neck, or soles. Scabies is usually spread through close contact. The female mite can survive away from the human for more than four days, so to prevent your reinfestation, your doctor may have told you to wash clothing, bed linens, and towels. It may be difficult to determine from where you got the scabies, because the itching usually starts about a month after the infestation. To be sure that your itch is caused by scabies, see your doctor, who will take and evaluate a specimen of the infected area so that he or she can prescribe appropriate treatment.

Q: *Does it hurt to have a mole removed?*
A: As with most surgical procedures, it is fear and anticipation of the procedure that causes the most concern. Removal of a mole usually is not very difficult. Your doctor will give you a local anesthetic, which can eliminate virtually all of the pain. In your consideration of surgery, you need to weigh the possible long-term effects of not treating the mole and consider all the treatment you would have to have if you developed a form of cancer because you ignored the problem. You should consult your health care provider if you have any questions about a mole, a wart, or any other skin problem.

15

Sleep Regulation for Children and Adults

Joanne Getsy, M.D.

We are not taught how to sleep, and most of us who do not have difficulty sleeping assume that it is easy to sleep. But for those who suffer from sleep disorders, fatigue and irritability are a part of daily life. This chapter deals specifically with children's sleeping problems; in the question-and-answer section I respond to questions about adults and sleep. This discussion may make you aware that you have a problem, and once you are able to identify it, you can begin to solve it.

Our sleep patterns begin when we are infants. Many children experience difficulty with their sleep, and most parents agree that this is one of the most troubling areas of parenthood. Because good sleep habits are formed so early in life, your child's sleep problems should be dealt with right away. Most can be remedied fairly easily with time, patience, and the right information.

Children and Sleep

Sleep is divided into *light,* *deep,* and *dream* sleep. These stages occur in regular intervals throughout the night. Children usually get most of their deep sleep early in the night (between 9 p.m. and midnight), but most of the dream and light sleep comes late, in the early hours of the morning. Newborns can spend more than half of their sleep in dream sleep, although it is not clear that they "dream" the way adults do. As the infant grows, he or she will have more deep sleep and less dream sleep.

Infants

Many parents marvel at how much their newborn baby sleeps during the first weeks of life. Soon this changes, and parents may become frustrated as their baby sleeps most of the day and stays up at night. Newborns sleep for sixteen to eighteen hours a day, usually in several two- to four-hour "naps," with one to two hours of wakefulness in between. They do not understand or sense night and day, so they function on a twenty-four-hour cycle for the first two months or so. Soon they begin to consolidate their sleep into longer sleep periods at night and shorter naps during the day. This is helped by environmental cues, such as light and dark, feeding time, and other activity in the house. By the age of approximately three months, babies should be able to sleep for at least five hours straight during the night (for example, from midnight to five a.m.). Their nutritional needs are such that they awaken to eat but should then be able to go back to sleep. Parents can encourage the consolidation of sleep into longer periods at night by keeping the nursery dark (use a small night light) and quiet, avoiding too much play and stimulation at night, and by not over- or underfeeding the baby during the night.

By age five or six months, most babies will sleep for longer periods at night, often up to eight hours without awaking. By age seven or eight months, many infants can sleep for nine to ten hours before awaking.

Napping

Once a baby has established a day/night cycle so that he or she is sleeping for longer periods (more than five uninterrupted hours) at night, he or she will begin to consolidate daytime sleep into approximately four naps during the day, each an hour or so long. As nighttime sleep increases, daytime sleep decreases. By the time an infant is sleeping for most of the night, he or she should be taking fewer daytime naps, perhaps two or three, each somewhat longer, up to two hours. Soon the infant sleeps all night (ten or eleven hours) and naps twice during the day. This should be achieved somewhere between ages seven and ten months. These naps should occur at approximately the same time every day. Babies should be allowed to nap in a comfortable, quiet location, preferably in their crib in a separate room. It is not usually necessary to be perfectly quiet while a baby sleeps because this will teach the baby to need absolute quiet in order to nap.

Nighttime Feedings

Infants need a great deal of nourishment early on, often needing to be fed every two or three hours, even at night. Once they reach age three months, however, most babies can skip a feeding in the middle of the night. By age six months, the majority of infants do not need to be fed during the night.

Nighttime Awakenings

Infants, like older children and adults, awaken briefly during the night. They should be able to go right back to sleep, as most adults do. Most adults, in fact, are not aware that they awaken periodically at night. We have learned to put ourselves back to sleep. The awakening is so brief that we usually do not recall it in the morning. Babies do the same thing. The difference is that some babies cannot put themselves back to sleep, so they may cry out for help. Mom or Dad comforts the baby and rocks or walks the infant to sleep again. This can go on indefinitely, until the child learns to go to sleep alone. Babies need to be allowed to fall asleep alone, without being cuddled or nursed or rocked, so that when they experience a normal, brief awakening at night, they will be able to go back to sleep without help from Mom or Dad.

Young Children

Sleep disturbances are remarkably common in children aged two through twelve. Indeed, it is perfectly normal for children to experience some difficulty sleeping at some point. Most of these problems will resolve themselves and do not need special medical attention. Some sleep problems can be associated with other diseases, however, and should be investigated.

Nightmares and Night Terrors

At some time we have all had *nightmares,* or disturbing dreams, that cause us to wake up frightened. Although we are frightened, we are aware of our surroundings and that we have just had a nightmare, and we are consolable. *Night terrors* are very different, however, and parents should not confuse them with nightmares. They are not dreams at all. During a night terror, a sleeping child suddenly begins screaming wildly, often sits upright in bed, cries, and is disoriented. He or she usually does not appear to recognize or respond to familiar people, even parents, and cannot be comforted or consoled. Several minutes may pass before the screaming child eventually tires and goes back to sleep. These episodes occur when the child is in very deep sleep, and their cause is unknown. After a nightmare, the child is awake and upset, but consolable. He or she calms down reasonably quickly and can recognize and respond to parents. The child experiencing a night terror, however, is actually still asleep, is very upset, is screaming or crying, does not recognize parents or others, and is not easily comforted. Children do not remember having night terrors the next morning. Fortunately, night terrors tend to go away with time and are uncommon after adolescence. In most children, they are not thought to be associated with any psychological disturbance.

Bedwetting (Enuresis)

Once young children are toilet-trained, most are able to stay dry at night, but some continue to wet during the night. Children with *primary enuresis* are not able to stay dry at night. Children with *secondary enuresis* are able to stay dry for months or years but later begin wetting at night. Both conditions are associated with many causes, and both need to be evaluated by a physician. In some instances, bedwetting is caused by an abnormality in the urinary system or by an infection of the kidneys or bladder. In other cases, it may be caused by the child's inability to sense the need to urinate, perhaps when in deep sleep. Also, the origin of bedwetting may be related to psychological problems or to stress of some type.

A parent should never scold a child for wetting the bed. Scolding usually adds to the child's shame and embarrassment and may lead to further wetting. A child who repeatedly wets the bed at night should be examined by the pediatrician or family doctor; the doctor might then refer the child to a specialist, such as a pediatric urologist.

Treatment of bedwetting depends on the cause. An abnormality or infection in the urinary system is treated with medication or, more rarely, with surgery. If a possible psychological cause is found, such as depression, anxiety, or stress, treatment includes counseling. Often, physicians are unable to find a specific reason for a child's bedwetting. Still, children with enuresis may be treated with behavioral techniques. The parents can wake the child once or twice at night to use the bathroom, or they can attach a small sensor to the child's underwear, which sounds to awaken the child when he or she wets. In some cases, your pediatrician may prescribe medication, and this can be very successful. In any case, children who wet the bed should be evaluated because the vast majority can be treated successfully.

Sleepwalking and Sleeptalking

Both sleepwalking and sleeptalking are reasonably common in young children. They typically occur during deep sleep, and the child does not remember the event in the morning. These curious behaviors do not usually represent any hidden psychological abnormality. Although they should be discussed with the child's doctor, seldom is any special sleep investigation needed. Parents should be aware, however, of the danger that sleepwalkers can get into. Sleepwalkers are actually asleep and are unaware of their surroundings. They have been known to walk into walls, fall down steps, even to go outside into traffic. Children who sleepwalk need to be protected from such dangers. Doors should be locked, gates may need to be used, and in some cases, the child may even need to be protected by an alarm, which sounds when he or she gets up.

Adolescents

Adolescence is a difficult time for children because their bodies go through dramatic changes. Their sleep patterns change, too, and will eventually evolve into those of an adult. During the years from puberty to the late teens, however, children seem to sleep endlessly, often twelve to fourteen hours a day. Adolescents typically adjust their sleep time, going to bed later and arising later, especially on weekends. Since teenagers often stay up late on school nights but still have to get up early, they become somewhat sleep deprived during the week but typically recover on the weekend, sleeping until noon. This is quite common and normal, although often frustrating for parents. These long sleep periods are thought to be necessary possibly because of the growth spurts occurring during adolescence. Parents can help teenagers by encouraging regular sleep schedules. Teens should not be allowed to "cheat" on their sleep by staying up late on school nights and then "catching up" on the weekends. Parents must keep in mind, however, that adolescents need more sleep than adults, and they should be allowed to sleep until they wake up naturally whenever possible, such as on the weekends and vacations. A reasonable bedtime for school nights and one for weekends should be agreed on by the teenager and the parents, one that allows enough sleep on a regular basis (at least eight hours of sleep per night during the week, more on the weekends).

Fortunately, most children do not have serious sleep problems, although most, from time to time, will have some minor difficulty. Problems with sleep should always be discussed with the child's doctor, who will help parents decide whether further referral is warranted. Sleep should be a pleasant experience for children. Parents can help them achieve a good attitude toward sleep by remembering that it is a skill to be learned and that it should never be used as a form of punishment.

About the Author

Dr. Joanne Getsy is an expert in the field of sleep disorders medicine. After graduating from Tufts Medical School in Boston in 1983, she went to the University of Pennsylvania, where she completed her internal medicine residency, as well as a fellowship in pulmonary disease. Dr. Getsy went on to study sleep disorders for two years before being named medical director of the Sleep Center at the Hospital of the University of Pennsylvania. She served in this capacity for three years before leaving to join the faculty of the Medical College of Pennsylvania.

QUESTIONS FOR THE DOCTOR

How much time do we spend sleeping and why do we sleep?
We spend one-third of our lives sleeping, yet few of us think about sleep until we have a problem with it. Sleep is a state of relaxation in which the sleeper, for the most part, is unaware of his or her surroundings. Sleep is defined scientifically by the activity of the brain. As one goes from wakefulness to sleep, the brain slows down, and this is reflected in the brain waves recorded at the scalp.

Every animal species that can be studied appears to sleep, or at least to have a period of inactivity similar to sleep. Most animals and humans sleep at roughly the same time period each night. Animals get enough sleep to be able to function normally the next day, but humans often "cheat" on the amount of sleep they get. It is clear, however, that we all need sleep.

I have heard there are "sleep stages." What are they?
Sleep is defined scientifically by the brain waves recorded by small electrodes, or sensors, that are glued or taped onto the scalp during an overnight sleep study. There are several different kinds of sleep, divided into "stages." *Stage 1* sleep is also called "transitional sleep," since it is the type of sleep that is between wakefulness and true sleep. People who are in Stage 1 sleep are sometimes able to hear things going on around them, but they are not fully alert. This is the sleep one goes into first when drifting off to sleep, and it is considered "light sleep."

Stage 2 sleep is also considered "light sleep," but it is slightly deeper than Stage 1. This is the kind of sleep one gets during a short afternoon nap. During Stage 2 sleep, people are not aware of their surroundings and they wake up afterward realizing that they have been asleep. The brain activity is somewhat slower than in Stage 1 sleep. People in Stage 2 sleep are still arousable without much difficulty. Adults spend most of their night in Stage 2 sleep.

Stage 3 and *Stage 4* sleep are considered "deep sleep." During these stages of sleep the brain slows down substantially, and people are difficult to arouse. These are both very satisfying, restful stages of sleep. Adults get most of our deep sleep during the first half of the night. When we deprive ourselves of sleep, then go to bed to recover, we recover deep sleep first, then lighter sleep later in the night. (Children get more deep sleep than do adults.) You can recognize deep sleep by how difficult it is to wake someone when they're in these deep stages of sleep.

The last stage of sleep is called *Rapid Eye Movement* (or REM) sleep. This is the dream sleep, the period of sleep when our brains are actively dreaming. The brain waves during REM sleep look almost like they do during wakefulness. This is the stage when we have our most complex dreams and nightmares. Although the brain is very active during REM sleep, the body is almost completely paralyzed.

The various sleep stages occur at regular times throughout the night. In general, adults get their Stage 3 and Stage 4 sleep (deep sleep) early in the night and get most of their REM sleep toward the second half of the night. REM sleep occurs every ninety minutes or so throughout the night. The first REM sleep period per night lasts only a few minutes, but each successive period gets longer. Thus, the longest period of REM sleep is early in the morning, just before getting up. Between REM periods, most of the night is spent in Stage 2 sleep.

Does the amount of sleep change as we age?
Infants spend a great deal of time sleeping, and more than half of their sleep can be REM sleep. By the time they are a few years old, sleep

begins to become consolidated into nighttime sleep, with an occasional daytime nap. Between ages two and twelve, children still get a large amount of deep sleep, but they get less REM than when they were infants. As much of one-third of a young child's night can be spent in deep sleep and approximately one-quarter in REM sleep. This pattern changes as the child grows, and by the early teens, the amount of both deep sleep and REM sleep starts to diminish. During adolescence, there is a period of time when more sleep is needed; this occurs during "growth spurts," and teenagers may spend as many as fourteen hours a day in bed, especially on weekends. This need for increased sleep appears to allow the teen to grow. Certain growth hormones are released by the body when the child is sleeping.

The amount of deep sleep and REM sleep continue to diminish, and by age eighteen or so, the adult sleep pattern has been reached. Adults spend more than half the night in Stage 2, very little (a few minutes) in Stage 1, approximately one-quarter of the night in Stages 3 and 4, and one-quarter in REM sleep. As as adult gets older, the amount of Stages 3 and 4 and REM sleep diminish, and Stage 2 occupies more of the night.

Older adults, over age sixty-five, often complain of difficulty sleeping. This difficulty becomes even more pronounced at older ages. Normal older adults spend less time in deep sleep and more in light sleep, thus feeling less rested when they awaken. In addition, older people tend to wake up more throughout the night, sometimes waking up to the slightest noise. Finally, the elderly tend to take more time to fall asleep than they did when they were younger. They also wake up earlier. This can be very frustrating, and the frustration can lead to further sleep loss. Such individuals sometimes have to nap in the afternoon to catch up on their sleep. This pattern of difficulty sleeping appears to be quite common in the elderly.

How much sleep do we need?

The amount of sleep one needs varies from person to person, but everyone needs to sleep. Most people need between seven and nine hours of sleep per night. There are people, however, who need only four to five hours of sleep nightly, and there are those who need as much as ten to twelve hours of sleep each night. The definition of "enough sleep" is the number of hours of sleep needed on a regular, nightly basis in order to feel alert and productive during the day, without the need for a daytime nap and without stimulants. If you are one of the lucky people who can function well on just a few hours of sleep, and you do not need to recover on the weekends, you are in the minority.

What most people do is "cheat" on their sleep, that is, they get less sleep than they actually need and then try to catch up later. For example, if a person needs eight hours of sleep to feel well but can get only six hours a night during the week, then he or she is cheating by two hours each night. By the end of the week, ten hours of sleep have been missed. This is called a "sleep debt," and it will continue to be accumulated until it is "paid back." Most people pay back the debt on the weekends, when they don't have to go to work. One can pay back less than the amount borrowed and still feel recovered. So, the person whose sleep debt is ten hours by the end of a work week typically pays back only a few hours of extra sleep on the weekend and feels fully recovered and ready to tackle another week.

The problem with cheating on sleep like this is that although one can recover on the weekends, there is a price to pay. That price is the poor performance many people have toward the end of a typical work week. Because so many people cheat on their sleep, most people are more tired toward the end of the week than they are in the beginning. As a result, more mistakes are made on Thursdays and Fridays than are made on Mondays and Tuesdays. More car accidents occur at the end of the week because people are tired and less attentive while driving. So, although it is possible for the body to recover from sleep loss, there is a serious price to pay.

Do a large number of people have difficulty sleeping?
Many people have difficulty. In a recent national survey, as many as three-quarters of those asked admitted to having an occasional problem with sleep. Most of us realize that without a good night's sleep our daytime functioning can be severely impaired.

How do doctors treat sleep disorders?
In order to study problems with sleep, special sleep centers have been established, staffed by specialists in the field. The evaluation usually begins with a consultation with one of the sleep specialists, who tries to understand the problem by asking questions and by having the patient fill out a questionnaire and perhaps a sleep diary. This is sometimes followed by an overnight sleep study. During this test, sensors are applied with special glue or tape to the head, face, chest, abdomen, and legs in order to record all activity during sleep. These monitors record brain waves, eye movements, muscle activity, breathing patterns, and oxygen level while the person is sleeping. In this way, specialists can try to uncover any problems you may be having with sleep and begin proper treatment.

What is insomnia?
When discussing insomnia, sleep experts separate the inability to fall asleep from the inability to stay asleep. That is, does the insomnia make

it difficult for a patient to fall asleep until very late or does the patient fall asleep but then wake up during the night? Also, we often distinguish *transient* (temporary) insomnia from *chronic,* long-standing insomnia.

Some medical disorders can lead to insomnia. For example, patients with hyperthyroidism (an overactive thyroid) may complain of the inability to sleep well. Also, diabetes, asthma, heart problems, ulcer disease, and some neurologic disorders can cause sleep disruption. Sometimes insomnia is caused by a specific sleep disorder; the following are three of the most common.

Delayed Sleep Phase Syndrome: This is a disorder in which the body's natural rhythm is off by a few hours and the person is not ready to go to bed until several hours later than the average person. These people are sometimes called "night owls." Generally, if left undisturbed, they go to bed very late, but then sleep until late into the morning and feel fine. The problem comes when such people have to get up early to go to work.

A person may be unable to fall asleep because he or she is trying to sleep when the body is not ready. This type of sleep disorder is quite common in teenagers. It can be adjusted so that the affected individual can be taught to go to bed at the correct time. One way to adjust the body's "clock" is to move the bedtime by a few hours each night. For example, if a person with the delayed sleep phase syndrome normally goes to bed at 3 A.M., we would change that bedtime to 5 A.M. on day number one. He or she then sleeps for their usual seven to eight hours and then gets up (this may require an alarm clock). The next night, the bedtime is changed to 7 A.M., and the person again sleeps for the usual seven to eight hours. The following night the bedtimme is at 9 A.M., and the next day at 11 A.M., and so on, each day allowing the person to sleep for his or her usual amount of time. In this way the bedtime is gradually advanced until the person is going to bed at 10 or 11 P.M. This type of therapy is called "chronotherapy" and is best done under the watchful eye of a sleep specialist.

Periodic Leg Movement Disorder: This is a sleep disorder characterized by frequent small leg twitches (often not felt by the patient) that cause the brain to wake up during the night. Sometimes the brain will be able to go right back to sleep, but other times it will not. This disorder is fairly common in older people, but it can occur at almost any age. It can be diagnosed only by an overnight sleep study. It is not caused by any serious neurologic or muscle disease and is reasonably easy to treat with medications.

Psychophysiologic Insomnia: This is a learned behavior that is possible to control and conquer with appropriate therapy. Typically, a bout of this type of insomnia begins with a particular stressful event, such as the loss of a job or an illness in the family. After the stress is gone, however, the difficulty sleeping persists and can even get worse. The person feels "out of control" and unable to get a good night's sleep. Every night is a bad one, and the person may begin to fear going to bed. If you think you may be suffering from psychophysiological insomnia, consult your physician.

How do physicians evaluate insomnia?

The first step in the evaluation of insomnia begins with a visit to a sleep specialist at the recommendation of your family physician. He or she will discuss your sleep history and may ask you to complete a questionnaire or a sleep diary. You may be asked to undergo an overnight sleep study in a sleep center so that the pattern of your sleep can be evaluated, and so that some of the disorders mentioned above can be looked for. If you are under a great deal of stress the sleep specialist may recommend that you see a psychologist or psychiatrist who specializes in sleep disorders to learn how to relax and get better sleep. The plan designed for an individual will depend on the result of the overall evaluation. If a medical disorder is suspected or diagnosed, further evaluation would be pursued. If a particular sleep disorder such as the periodic leg movement disorder is diagnosed, this would be treated with medications. If, after a complete evaluation, the sleep physician believes that the insomnia may be due to factors such as stress, anxiety, work, etc., he or she may opt to begin a treatment plan that includes sleep relaxation techniques, behavior modification, or more intense therapy.

What can I do to improve my sleep?

Make sleep a priority.   Remember that sleep is necessary, and if you are cheating on your sleep chances are your cheating will catch up with you. Schedule your day and evening to allow time at night for sleep!

Keep a regular bedtime and wake time.   Keeping regular sleeping hours helps regulate your body rhythm, and will often help you to fall asleep more readily. This may also include keeping regular hours on weekends until you are sleeping better. Go to bed at the same hour every night, and set an alarm to get up at roughly the same time each day.

Exercise.   Studies have shown that regular exercise deepens sleep. It is best to exercise in the morning, but if this is not possible, be sure your exercise is completed before 7:00 P.M. to avoid being kept awake from the stimulation from the exercise.

Make your bedroom comfortable.   Your bedroom should be conducive to sleep, and it should be comfortable, soothing, and dark. Stress-provoking items such as those related to work and bills should not be in the bedroom.

Eat a light snack.   Hunger will disturb sleep, but so will a big meal before bedtime. Eat dinner several hours before retiring, and if you are hungry at bedtime, have a light snack.

Avoid caffeine and nicotine.   Both disturb sleep. Do not drink any caffeine-containing drinks within six hours of bedtime. Cigarettes are harmful in many ways; that nicotine may contribute to insomnia is just one of the negatives. If you cannot quit smoking, avoid cigarettes for at least two hours before bedtime.

Drink no alcohol before bedtime.   Many people think that a "nightcap" helps one sleep, but it can actually disrupt sleep and worsen insomnia. It is best to avoid drinking alcohol within a few hours of going to bed.

Relax.   Give yourself time to unwind before going to bed. Stop working at least two hours before bedtime, and take some relaxation time to prepare for sleep.

Develop a routine for bed.   Begin relaxing and preparing for bed about two hours before bedtime. Get into a routine that helps you get ready to fall asleep.

Don't be a clock-watcher.   When you are trying to fall asleep, or if you wake up in the middle of the night, *don't* look at the clock and worry about what time it is. Turn the clock away from you, or put it somewhere else in the room where you cannot see it. The anxiety of clock-watching makes it more difficult to fall asleep.

Don't try to force sleep.   If you cannot fall asleep within a short amount of time, get up and do something else like reading, watching television, or listening to soothing music. Go back to bed when you feel sleepy.

Try another room.   If you find it difficult to sleep in your usual bedroom, try moving to another room. Sometimes the insomnia is associated with your bedroom, and you *expect* not to sleep in this room. Try another room, *expect* to sleep, and you *will* be able to sleep.

I am a sleepwalker. Why do people walk and talk when they sleep?
These two disorders are quite common in children and usually disappear by the time the child is an adolescent. They occur during sleep Stages 2, 3, and 4, but not during REM sleep. Sleeptalking is harmless, for the most part, and usually does not require much evaluation, unless the child has a neurologic or seizure disorder or appears to act strangely during sleep.

Make the child's physician aware of the sleeptalking and he or she will decide if any evaluation is necessary. Sleepwalking is common and not necessarily a sign of an underlying disorder, but it sometimes requires an evaluation (this, too, should be decided by the child's physician). The main problem with sleepwalking is that the sleepwalker can injure himself or herself. The person is actually asleep while walking around and is unaware of his or her surroundings. Therefore, he or she can walk out onto a busy street, turn on the oven, or do other dangerous activities and be completely unaware. Sometimes barriers or doors have to be installed to keep the sleepwalker in a safe environment to avoid harm.

Sleepwalking is very common in children, but not common in adults. Children should outgrow it by the time of adolescence; if they do not, a formal investigation may be necessary. Sleepwalking in adults can sometimes be a sign of an underlying neurologic disorder and should be evaluated by a sleep specialist. Sleepwalking can be controlled with medication if necessary.

My child wets the bed at least once a week. Why does she do this?

Bedwetting, also called enuresis, is reasonably common in young children. Specialists sometimes separate bedwetting into "primary" and "secondary." *Primary bedwetting* refers to the bedwetting that occurs as an infant. It continues into adulthood, with the child never really having a period of time when he or she stayed dry at night. *Secondary betwetting* refers to bedwetting that comes after the child has learned to stay dry. Both need to be evaluated. Most family physicians and pediatricians are familiar with bedwetting and are the first people to see for advice. The physician may refer the child to a specialist, such as a pediatric urologist, who deals with the urinary system of children. These specialists can determine whether a formal evaluation for a urinary problem is necessary. Sometimes bedwetting is due to a structural abnormality of the urinary system, though other times no structural urological problem can be identified—in this case, the bedwetting may be due to psychological or family issues. This does *not* mean that the child has a severe psychological disturbance. More commonly, there is no obvious problem; in fact, the child is often not aware of any problems. He or she may be well-adjusted, happy, and under no particular stress and may still wet the bed.

The treatment for enuresis depends on the cause. For some children, medication or correction of a structural abnormality may be necessary. For others, behavioral techniques (with or without medications) might be used to teach the child to stay dry at night. For example, there are some useful "alarms" that can be used during sleep to teach the child to awaken when he or she begins to wet. These are safe, harmless, and often very effective. One type consists of little paper strips that are placed into the child's underpants before going to bed. When a drop of urine touches the strip, a noise is generated. This wakes the child and reminds him or her to go to the bathroom to empty the bladder. He or she then places a new strip in a clean pair of underwear and goes back to sleep.

There are different types of behavioral techniques, all designed to teach the child to stay dry by himself or herself. These methods avoid the embarrassment of having to ask for help and the shame of wetting the bed. Whatever type of therapy is prescribed, most children outgrow bed-wetting by the time of adolescence and are able to stay dry at night for the rest of their lives.

What is narcolepsy?

Narcolepsy is a disorder of extreme sleepiness, usually starting in the teenage years or early twenties. It is characterized by severe, periodic daytime sleepiness, which often forces the person afflicted to take one or several naps during the day. The cause is unknown, but it appears to run in families. At times the diagnosis is not made for many years, and patients may not know they have it until they are much older.

The abnormality in narcolepsy involves changes with Rapid Eye Movement sleep. Patients with narcolepsy get an overwhelming feeling of sleepiness during the day, even if they have slept for a substantial time the night before. When they nap, they go into REM sleep within a few minutes. When most of us nap, we achieve Stage 2, or maybe even Stage 3 sleep, but we do not have REM sleep. Narcoleptics frequently have REM sleep during naps. Sometimes they dream when they nap. Afterwards, they wake feeling refreshed, as though their body needed a short period of REM sleep to feel better. Narcoleptics are otherwise completely normal, intelligent people who have no known neurologic problem associated with the narcolepsy. They sometimes have other symptoms that accompany the sleepiness. One is *cataplexy,* which refers to the loss of muscle tone or to the feeling of being completely or partially paralyzed when excited or upset. In extreme cases, patients with narcolepsy may actually fall to the ground after an emotional event.

Another symptom accompanying narcolepsy is *sleep paralysis,* which refers to waking up and feeling completely paralyzed. This occurs when one wakes up in the middle of REM sleep. Although the brain might wake up, the body can still be paralyzed. Although this may happen occasionally to people without narcolepsy, it can happen frequently to narcoleptics. Finally, some narcolepsy patients experience what are called *hypnogogic hallucinations.* These are dreamlike events that occur as narcoleptics are falling asleep. Experts believe these events happen when a narcoleptic falls into REM sleep quickly and begins to have a dream although they are barely asleep.

How do doctors discover if someone has narcolepsy?

The diagnosis of narcolepsy is made with a formal sleep study, which includes the overnight sleep test as well as a daytime test called a *multiple sleep latency test*. This test consists of a series of scheduled naps during the day, during which the brain waves and other parameters are measured to see if REM sleep is achieved during the naps. With the history of persistent, severe daytime sleepiness and the demonstration of REM sleep during daytime naps, the doctor can establish the diagnosis of narcolepsy.

The treatment of this disorder involves a combination of medication and scheduled naps. Stimulants are used to help keep people with narcolepsy awake during the day. This allows them to function normally, maintain jobs, drive automobiles safely, and so forth. Some patients must remain on medications indefinitely, in order to keep awake during the day. Still, this is a treatable disorder, and patients can lead normal, productive lives.

My husband was told he has sleep apnea. What is it?

Obstructive sleep apnea syndrome refers to a disorder in which there is the cessation of breathing during sleep. It occurs primarily, but not exclusively, in middle-aged overweight men. But it can also occur in children, women, and people of normal body weight. It usually afflicts people who snore. In this disorder, the throat actually collapses during sleep, making it impossible for air to pass into the lungs. The person stops snoring as the throat is collapsed because no air gets through. This typically goes on for ten to twenty seconds, but it can last as long as one to two minutes. Finally, the brain realizes the person is not breathing. At that point, the brain arouses just enough to cause the throat to open. This produces a loud snore, snort, or choking sensation, followed by the usual snoring. This period of time, when there is no airflow, is called an *apnea*. Apneas can occur up to hundreds of times throughout the night, although the afflicted person typically has no idea that this is happening. It usually takes a bed partner to notice the apneas. The patient may notice that he or she is falling asleep at inappropriate times or is tired during the day, often to the point of needing to take naps. This is because sleep is usually very light and is interrupted repeatedly by the apneas. The brain is constantly being disturbed during sleep because it has to be stimulated each time the person stops breathing in order to restart the breathing. As a result, sleep is of poor quality and the person feels tired the next day.

In addition to the sleepiness during the day, sleep apnea produces a number of serious side effects. During an apnea, when there is no air movement into the lungs, the oxygen level in the blood falls. The result can be a strain on the heart, causing high blood pressure and heart disease. Furthermore, there is evidence that untreated sleep apnea can lead to strokes in some people. By far the most common and the earliest sign of sleep apnea is sleepiness during the day, which can lead to automobile accidents, poor performance at work, irritability, and trouble remembering the simplest detail.

Obstructive sleep apnea is more common in men, especially men who are overweight. Researchers believe this is due, in part, to the deposition of fat within the throat, rendering the throat more narrow and thus more likely to collapse when relaxed during sleep. In addition, the fat deposited within the neck itself can contribute to the collapse of the throat. For example, sleep apnea is more common in men with collar size above sixteen and one-half. Almost anyone can get sleep apnea if there is some problem with the upper airway, however. For example, it can occur because of a deviated nasal septum, large tonsils, or adenoids. It can occur in people with small jaws or large tongues. It can even happen to children, especially those with large tonsils.

The diagnosis of apnea is suspected in a person who snores and is tired during the day or evening. This diagnosis is often reinforced by the bed partner, who may notice periods of time when the person is not breathing during sleep. An overnight sleep study is used to help diagnose obstructive sleep apnea. The sensors that are applied serve to indicate when the person stops breathing and show how low the person's oxygen level falls. The total number of times a person stops breathing over the course of the night is counted and then divided by the number of hours of sleep to give an "apnea index," the number of apneas per hour of sleep. In general, more than seven or eight apneas per hour is significant. People with very severe obstructive sleep apnea may stop breathing over fifty times per hour, sometimes as many as one hundred times per hour.

The treatment of this disease depends on the suspected cause. If there is a defined abnormality, such as large tonsils or adenoids or a deviated nasal septum, sometimes surgical correction is the answer. For the vast majority of patients, however, the treatment is twofold. Certainly, they need to lose weight, and many times this causes the sleep apnea to disappear. In the meantime, though, they are at risk for further problems and should be treated with a device called the nasal CPAP, the treatment of choice for this disorder. CPAP stands for "continuous positive airway pressure." This device consists of a specially designed air compressor that blows air through a tube into a mask worn over the nose or through a set of soft plastic plugs that fit into the nostrils. The machine is set to the correct pressure so that air is blown through the tubing, into the nose, and down the back of the throat. In this way, the air "blows" the throat open with just enough pressure to distend the airway so that it cannot collapse during sleep. With the use of the CPAP, the throat stays open, breathing is normal, and snoring is completely gone. The person sleeps peacefully and gets the refreshing, deep sleep that he or she has not had for months or even years. Some people feel better after only a few nights of using the nasal CPAP. The device must be worn every night during sleep, but is not worn during the day unless the person decides to take a nap. The nasal CPAP requires a prescription from a physician. The patient must first undergo an overnight sleep study. The CPAP must be started during a sleep study so that the correct pressure or amount of air can be determined, and then prescribed. The CPAP is then used nightly until the patient is able to lose enough weight so that the sleep apnea disappears. If he or she cannot lose weight (or does not need to), the nasal CPAP can be used indefinitely. There are hundreds of thousands of people currently using CPAP. It is a safe, effective treatment for obstructive sleep apnea.

For some patients, obstructive apneas occur only when they are sleeping on their backs, not when they are on their sides. This can only be proven during an overnight sleep study. If it is shown that the apneas depend on position, one very simple therapy is used to keep the person off his or her back, the "tennis ball" technique. This involves placing a tennis ball in the back of the pajamas, between the shoulder blades. This can be accomplished by sewing a pocket into the pajama top or t-shirt in the area between the shoulder blades and then placing a tennis ball into the pocket, or you can place a tennis ball in a sock and pin or sew the sock to the pajama top so that it rests in the back. Because the tennis ball gets in the way when the sleeping person tries to lie on his or her back, it is very uncomfortable and the person will naturally roll onto his or her side or stomach, alleviating the apneas.

Other possible treatments for obstructive sleep apnea include devices that fit in the mouth. These oral devices, made of a plastic material, look like the mouthguards boxers put in their mouths before fights. The devices for sleep apnea are smaller, however, and are specially fitted to each patient's mouth. They act to bring the lower jaw and tongue slightly forward. This opens the area in the back of the throat. Oral devices work for only some patients with sleep apnea. They should be prescribed by a physician who specializes in sleep disorders, after careful evaluation and sleep testing. A repeat sleep study with the oral device in place should be performed to make sure that the device abolishes all of the sleep apnea.

For some people with obstructive sleep apnea, surgery is an alternative to nasal CPAP, especially for patients who are not overweight. For these people, a careful evaluation by an ear, nose, and throat surgeon may demonstrate an abnormality in the nose or back of the throat that might be corrected with surgery (the most obvious example is that of large tonsils and adenoids). A surgery known as uvulopalatopharyngoplasty (UPPP) is often performed for obstructive sleep apnea. In this surgery, the uvula, soft palate, tonsils, and excess fatty tissue in the back of the throat are all removed in an attempt to open up the throat and prevent obstructive apnea from occurring.

UPPP works for only a small percentage of patients, and it should be performed only by an ear, nose, and throat surgeon with a special understanding of and expertise in the field of sleep disorders. Patients who are more than thirty pounds overweight do not usually respond well to this surgery and often still need nasal CPAP afterwards. For this reason, overweight patients who do not have a defined abnormality in their airway, such as large tonsils or adenoids, should use the twofold approach of losing weight and using nasal CPAP as their first line of therapy. Only after weight loss should these patients have an upper-airway surgery such as the UPPP, because, for thin patients or for patients of normal body weight, the UPPP can sometimes be very successful. There are also some special jaw surgeries that are performed by oral surgeons with special training that may work for some apnea patients. In general, patients with obstructive sleep apnea should consult a certified sleep specialist to get advice about which therapy is most suitable for them.

I am tired of my husband's snoring. Why is this such a problem?
Snoring is a very common problem, especially in men. Approximately 40 percent of men and 25 percent of women of age thirty snore. By age sixty, the percentages increase to 60 percent and 40 percent, respectively. This means that a great number of people snore. The severity of snoring may vary, but some people are able to produce sounds that are loud enough to keep the entire family awake. In general, snoring is more a nuisance than a true sleep disorder. It seldom bothers the person making the noise, but it can ruin a marriage when the spouse can no longer sleep in the same bed because of the noise.

There is some recent evidence that snoring may be associated with high blood pressure (hypertension) and, perhaps, with heart disease; this is especially true for someone with obstructive sleep apnea syndrome (see above). Snoring should be evaluated if the person has hypertension or heart disease, if the person is tired during the day, if the noise is disruptive to the bed partner, or if the bed partner has seen or heard the person stop breathing during sleep. In these cases, an overnight sleep study might be necessary to check for obstructive sleep apnea syndrome. It is important to diagnose apnea because it is associated with more side effects than is simple snoring.

What can be done about snoring?

The treatment for snoring depends on a number of factors. For example, if an overnight sleep study shows obstructive sleep apnea, review the treatment options discussed above and consult your physician. If there is no sleep apnea, just loud snoring, treatment is slightly different. If the snorer is overweight, weight loss can be an important part of treatment. For many people, losing weight may cause the snoring to disappear completely, but, more commonly, it becomes softer and more tolerable for the bed partner. The oral devices mentioned above for sleep apnea work well for snoring, too. Finally, surgery is available for snoring, although this type of surgery is best done by a surgeon with special expertise in sleep disorders. The "tennis ball" technique described for sleep apnea can be extremely effective for some snorers, sometimes resolving the problem easily. This method may be tried by almost anyone. It is an inexpensive, effective therapy. Finally, nasal CPAP may be used to try to abolish snoring.

My husband wakes up three to four times a night to urinate. Why isn't he sleeping as well as he used to?

Your husband should be examined by his doctor to see if his prostate is enlarged. Men with enlarged prostates often have to urinate several times during the night. Frequent urination and getting up at night to urinate are common symptoms of prostatic enlargement. Also consider how much fluid your husband drinks before he goes to bed or try to recall if he has had a problem with his kidneys in the past; both may be related to frequent urination.

My doctor doesn't know much about sleep disorders. Do you get any courses on sleep in medical school?

Most medical schools teach only the basics, because until now there has not been a great understanding of sleep disorders. Now, however, more specialists are starting to stress the need for educating physicians about the importance of good sleep hygiene, as well as about sleep disorders such as obstructive sleep apnea, narcolepsy, and insomnia. If your doctor cannot help you with a sleep problem, ask him or her to refer you to a sleep specialist. There are many well-trained sleep disorder specialists who are able to help you and your family sleep better.

16

Voice Disorders

Robert Thayer Sataloff, M.D., D.M.A.

The human voice is extraordinary. It is capable of conveying not only complex thought but also subtle emotion. In an instant, it can communicate the terror of a scream or the beauty of a song. Although humankind has appreciated the uniqueness and power of the human voice for centuries, only in the last few years have we begun to understand how the voice works, and how to care for it.

Anatomy of the Throat

It is beyond the scope of this chapter to go into great detail about the anatomy of the throat, but a few brief points need to be made. The *larynx* (voice box) is essential to normal voice production, although it is possible to produce voice even without a larynx; for example, in patients who have undergone laryngectomy (removal of the larynx) for cancer. The voice depends as well on other parts of the anatomy. The muscles of the abdomen and back, in addition to the rib cage, lungs, throat, oral cavity, and nose, all perform important functions in voice production. In addition, virtually all parts of the body play some role in voice production and may be responsible for voice problems. Consider that even a sprained ankle can affect the voice by altering posture and thereby impairing abdominal muscle function, which could result in vocal inefficiency, weakness, and hoarseness.

The larynx is composed of four basic units: skeleton, intrinsic mus-

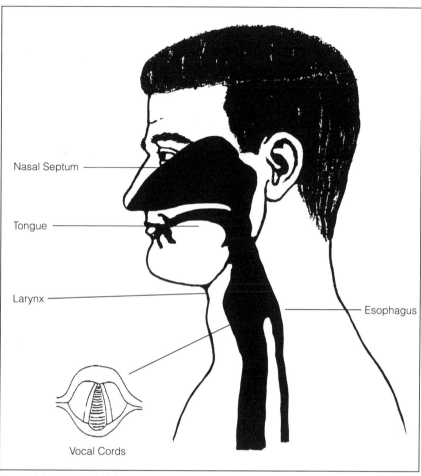

Critical Anatomy of Voice

cles, extrinsic muscles, and mucosa. The most important parts of the *laryngeal skeleton* are the several kinds of cartilage, which are connected to specialized muscles called the *intrinsic muscles* of the larynx. On each side, one of these muscles (the *thyroarytenoid,* or *vocalis,* muscle) extends behind the "Adam's apple," forming the body of the *vocal folds* (popularly called the *vocal cords*). The vocal folds act as the oscillator, or voice source, of the vocal tracts. The intrinsic muscles alter the position, shape, and tension of the vocal folds, bringing them together or apart or stretching them by increasing tension. Another intrinsic muscle, the *cricothyroid muscle,* helps control volume and pitch. Structures called the "false vocal folds" are located above the vocal folds and, unlike the true vocal folds, do not make contact during normal speaking or singing. The extrinsic muscles can be felt under the skin of the neck. They maintain vertical laryngeal position and influence indirectly the intrinsic muscles.

But there is more to a good voice than the voice box, however. Abdominal muscles and related structures can serve as a power source for the voice. Singers and actors refer to the entire power source complex as their "support" or "diaphragm." Actually, the anatomy of support for voice is complicated and not completely understood, but it is quite clear that deficiencies in support are frequently responsible for voice dysfunction.

Medical Care of Voice Disorders

Until the 1980s, most physicians caring for patients with voice disorders asked only a few basic questions, such as: How long have you been hoarse? Do you smoke? The physician's ear was the sole "instrument" used routinely to assess voice quality and function. Visual examination of the vocal folds was restricted to looking through a mirror placed inside the mouth, using regular light, or to direct *laryngoscopy* (examination of the interior of the larynx, with anesthesia in the operating room, using an instrument called a *laryngoscope*). Treatment was generally limited to medicines for infection or inflammation, or to surgery for bumps or masses. Occasionally, "voice therapy" was recommended, but the specific nature of the therapy was not well controlled and the results were often disappointing. The standard of practice has changed dramatically in the last ten years.

Good medical diagnosis in all fields often hinges on the physician's asking the right questions and listening carefully to the answers. This process is known as "taking a history." The patient relates all the facts that he or she can recall regarding previous illnesses, infections, injuries, hospitalizations, surgeries, and so on. The physician's use of a patient's medical history to help diagnose problems of the larynx was the first major change in medical care for voice problems. Problems outside the larynx often cause voice dysfunction in people whose vocal folds appear fairly normal, and who would have received no effective medical care a few years ago.

Factors and Conditions Affecting the Voice

People with voice problems sometimes complain of "hoarseness" or "laryngitis." *Laryngitis,* caused by a swollen, inflamed larynx, may result in hoarseness. *Hoarseness,* when your voice sounds coarse or scratchy, is caused most commonly by abnormalities on the vibratory margin of the vocal folds. These abnormalities may include swelling, roughness from inflammation, growths, scarring, or anything that interferes with symmetric, periodic vocal fold vibration. Such abnormalities produce turbulence in the air passing through or over the folds, which we perceive as hoarseness. *Breathiness* is caused by lesions or conditions that keep the vocal folds from closing completely, including paralysis of one or both vocal folds, cricoarytenoid joint injury or arthritis, vocal fold masses, or atrophy of the vocal fold tissues. These abnormalities permit air to escape when the vocal folds are supposed to be tightly closed. We hear this air leak as breathiness.

Many factors must be investigated in anyone with a voice complaint. *Age* affects the voice significantly, especially during childhood and old age. In geriatric patients, vocal unsteadiness, loss of range, and voice fatigue may be associated with typical physiologic aging changes, such as *vocal fold atrophy.* In routine speech, such vocal changes allow a person to be identified as "old" even over the telephone. Among singers, these changes are typically associated with flat pitch and a "wobble."

Recent evidence has shown, however, that many of these acoustic phenomena are not caused by irreversible aging changes. Rather, they may be consequences of poor respiratory and abdominal muscle condition, which undermines the power source of the voice. In this case, the medical history usually reveals that the patient engages in minimal aerobic exercise and suffers shortness of breath when climbing stairs. With appropriate conditioning of the body and the voice, many of the characteristics associated with vocal aging can be eliminated.

The amount of *voice use* and *training* also affects voices. Inquiry into vocal habits frequently reveals correctable causes for voice difficulties. Extensive untrained speaking under adverse environmental circumstances, for example, is a syndrome common among stock traders, sales people, restaurant personnel, and people who speak over the telephone in noisy offices. Many suspect that President Bill Clinton suffers from this syndrome. These problems are worsened by habits that impair the mechanics of voice production, such as sitting with poor posture and bending the neck to hold a telephone against one shoulder. Subconscious efforts to overcome these impediments often produce enough voice abuse to cause vocal fatigue, hoarseness, and even nodules (callous-like growths, usually on both vocal folds). Eliminating these habits usually solves the problem; even the nodules disappear. The trauma associated with voice abuse may also cause other vocal fold masses including *cysts* (fluid-filled masses) and *polyps* (soft tissue growth, usually on one side). Cysts and polyps frequently do not respond to voice therapy and often require surgical treatment.

Exposure to *environmental irritants* is a well-recognized cause of voice dysfunction. Smoke, dehydration, pollution, and allergens may produce hoarseness, frequent throat clearing, and voice fatigue. These problems can generally be eliminated easily by avoiding irritants, medication, or simply by breathing through the nose rather than the mouth, since the nose warms, humidifies, and filters incoming air.

The harmful effects of tobacco smoke on the vocal folds have been known for many years. Smoking not only causes chronic irritation but also can result in changes to the cell layer covering the vocal fold. The cells change in appearance, becoming more and more different from normal cells; eventually, they begin to pile up on each other rather than line up in an orderly fashion. They grow rapidly without restraint and invade surrounding tissues. This change in laryngeal tissue is called *squamous cell carcinoma,* or cancer of the larynx.

The voice depends so heavily on constant breath support that it should not be surprising that even subtle *respiratory problems* can result in voice dysfunction. For example, we have only recently recognized a form of exercise-induced asthma precipitated by the "exercise" of singing or speaking. Frequently, patients with this problem are unaware of their condition. When it is corrected and their ability to maintain a controlled airstream returns, however, the vocal problems disappear.

Gastrointestinal disorders commonly cause voice complaints. The sphincter that controls the opening between the stomach and esophagus is notoriously weak. In *gastroesophageal reflux laryngitis,* stomach acid rises into the throat, allowing droplets of the irritating gastric juices to come in contact with the vocal folds, or even to enter the lungs. Common symptoms are hoarseness, especially in the morning, prolonged vocal warm-up time, bad breath, and a dry or "coated" mouth. People with this disorder typically do not have heartburn.

Hormonal problems also have marked vocal effects, primarily because fluid accumulates in the vocal folds and alters their vibrations. Mild hypothyroidism typically causes a muffled sound, a slight loss of range, and vocal sluggishness. Some women experience similar symptoms in pregnancy, during use of oral contraceptives (in about 5 percent of women), or for a few days prior to menses. Women who experience premenstrual loss of vocal efficiency, endurance, and range tend toward vocal fold hemmorhage (bleeding), which can permanently alter the voice.

The use of various *foods and drugs* may affect the voice, too. Some medications may even ruin a voice permanently, especially androgenic hormones, such as those given to women with endometriosis. Some more common drugs also have adverse vocal effects, but these effects are usually temporary. Antihistamines cause dryness, increased throat clearing, and irritation, and they often aggravate hoarseness. Aspirin's anticlotting properties contribute to vocal fold hemorrhages. The propellant in inhalers often produces laryngitis. Many other medications cause similar problems. Some foods may also be responsible for voice complaints in people with normal vocal folds. The casein in milk products is particularly troublesome to some people because it increases and thickens mucosal secretions.

A history of problems elsewhere in the body must also be considered when physicians are trying to determine the cause of a voice disorder. For example, because voice function relies on complex brain and nervous system interactions, even slight *neurological dysfunction* may cause voice abnormalities. Voice impairment is often the first symptom of serious diseases such as myasthenia gravis, multiple sclerosis, or Parkinson's disease. Even seemingly unrelated problems—like the sprained ankle mentioned earlier—can reveal the true cause of voice dysfunction, especially in a singer, actor, or speaker with great vocal demands. Proper posture is important to optimal function of the abdomen and chest, which is necessary to avoid compensatory vocal strain, leading to hoarseness and voice fatigue. Naturally, a history of laryngeal injury or surgery raises concerns about the vocal fold; but a history of interference with the power source through abdominal or chest surgery may be just as important in understanding the development and treatment of vocal problems. *Psychological disturbances* are also commonly reflected in the voice, and they may be the sole cause of severe voice abnormalities.

Treatment of Voice Disorders

Following a thorough examination of the patient's medical history, a physical examination, and a clinical voice laboratory analysis, it is usually possible for the physician to arrive at an accurate explanation for voice dysfunction. Treatment depends on the etiology (the cause and development), of course. Fortunately, because technology has improved voice medicines, the need for laryngeal surgery has diminished.

Many other medical conditions require the use of prescription drugs, but these medications must be used with caution because many of them have adverse side effects that alter voice function. For example, antihistamines cause drying that can lead to hoarseness and cough. Many medicines for neurological, psychological, and respiratory conditions cause tremor that can be heard in the voice. Consequently, close collaboration is required among all specialists involved in the patient's care to be certain that treatment of one causal condition does not produce a secondary dysfunction that is also deleterious to the voice. When the underlying problem is corrected properly, the voice usually improves; but collaborative treatment by a team of specialists is most desirable to insure good general and vocal health and to optimize voice function.

Voice abuse through technical dysfunction (misuse or abuse of the voice) is an extremely common source of hoarseness, vocal weakness, pain, and other complaints. Now that the systemic components of voice function are better understood, techniques have been developed to rehabilitate and train the voice both in speech and in singing. *Voice therapy* improves breathing and abdominal support, decreases excess muscle activity in the larynx and neck, optimizes the mechanics of transglottal airflow, and maximizes the contributions of resonance cavities. It also teaches *vocal hygiene*, including techniques to eliminate voice strain and abuse, to maintain hydration and mucosal function, to mitigate the effects of smoke and other environmental irritants, and to optimize vocal and general health.

There have been dramatic advances in voice medicine in the 1980s and 1990s. Some of these are, for example, more thorough history-taking to assess problems throughout the body that may be reflected in the voice; better physical examination with voice performance assessment and new instructions for laryngeal visualization; slow-motion assessment of the vocal folds, using video to look at movement; voice quantification in the voice laboratory, in which actual sounds are measured and interpreted; and much better treatment of all voice disorders. Nevertheless, prevention is still the best medicine against problems with the larynx. A great many voice problems are preventable through patient education and voice hygiene, and through voice training that prepares the voice to sustain the rigors of daily use.

About the Author

Dr. Robert Thayer Sataloff is professor of otolaryngology at Jefferson Medical College in Philadelphia and is on the faculty of the Academy of Vocal Arts and the Curtis Institute of Music. He is the author of over two hundred publications, including ten textbooks. He is also a professional singer, singing teacher, and choral conductor.

Dr. Sataloff's medical practice is limited to care of the professional voice, and to neurotology (microsurgery of the ear and ear-brain interface).

QUESTIONS FOR THE DOCTOR

Q: *I notice that I have been having a great deal of difficulty swallowing during the past few months. First it started out with solid foods, but it seems to be progressing to liquids. I'm having more difficulty swallowing as the weeks go on. Is this a potential problem? What could be causing this?*

A: It is very important for you to have this problem checked out by your physician. There are a number of conditions that could be causing it, but the most serious is cancer of the esophagus or another form of cancer that could be narrowing the space of the tube that goes from your mouth to your stomach. People with cancer of the esophagus often notice that they have this difficulty swallowing. Over time this becomes apparent with softer and softer foods. Cancer of the esophagus can be treated, but it needs to be diagnosed early. There are other things that could be causing this problem, including a *stricture* (narrowing) or even a foreign body; however, cancer is a major concern. The examination of your throat is relatively easy to do. You should consult your doctor whenever you experience hoarseness, pain, or difficulty swallowing.

Q: *I have consistent postnasal drip. Is this bad for my voice?*

A: Yes, it can be bad for your voice because of the irritation to your throat caused by the postnasal drip. A sensation of postnasal drip can also be caused by reflux of acid. Sinus fluid is a caustic irritant. Many times physicians see patients who have sore throats due to irritation from sinus fluid or stomach acid. Check with your doctor to see if he or she can suggest something you can do to eliminate your sinus problems.

Q: *I have heard that lung cancer can affect the voice. Is that true?*
A: The *recurrent laryngeal nerve,* which can be damaged by cancer, can cause hoarseness. Thus hoarseness in the voice can be a sign of lung or other forms of cancer.

Q: *I get canker sores almost every other month, and they make it difficult to talk and eat. Is there anything I can do about them?*
A: *Recurrent aphthous stomatitis* is a condition characterized by recurrent painful ulcerations, or canker sores, that can occur in almost any area inside the mouth, extending to the inside of the lips. There are many suspected causes, but no one is quite sure what the exact cause is. Ulcerative colitis, Crohn's disease, and vitamin deficiencies may be associated with the problem, and at one time it was thought that they were caused by a virus. This has recently been disputed. Aphthous stomatitis is more common in women. Canker sores appear as single or multiple shallow ulcerations that are white in the center and red around the outside. Most treatments for canker sores take seven to fourteen days to work, but these sores go away on their own in seven to fourteen days anyway. The best treatment, however, is avoidance of spicy, acidic, or salty foods, as well as sharp and hard foods. Cuts on the inside of the mouth can lead to increased ulcer formation. Consult your doctor about using a mixture of Benadryl and Kaopectate in equal parts as a mouth rinse four to six times a day.

Q: *I am a seventeen-year-old girl and guys say my voice is sexy because it is so raspy. My doctor says I have a polyp. What should I do?*
A: In the long run the polyp can cause serious difficulty, including hoarseness. I suggest that you see your doctor and have it treated. You need not be frightened; treatment does not always mean surgery. In many cases, the only treatment needed is voice therapy and rest to improve the situation.

Q: *I am a stutterer. Is there anything that can help me?*
A: Yes. Many people have been able to use techniques successfully to control and even to stop stuttering. Famous stutterers who have done this include James Earl Jones (employing a deep, breathy voice) and Bruce Willis. You should ask your otolaryngologist or family physician for help in locating a speech specialist in your area.